AF738965

Physical Therapy for Gastrointestinal Disorders

Jaime Ruiz-Tovar • Ana Martín-Nieto
Editors

Physical Therapy for Gastrointestinal Disorders

Springer

Editors
Jaime Ruiz-Tovar
San Juan de Dios Foundation
Madrid, Spain

Department of Health Sciences, San Juan de Dios School of Nursing and Physical Therapy
Comillas Pontifical University
Madrid, Spain

Ana Martín-Nieto
San Juan de Dios Foundation
Madrid, Spain

Department of Health Sciences, San Juan de Dios School of Nursing and Physical Therapy
Comillas Pontifical University
Madrid, Spain

ISBN 978-3-031-83650-3 ISBN 978-3-031-83651-0 (eBook)
https://doi.org/10.1007/978-3-031-83651-0

© The Editor(s) (if applicable) and The Author(s), under exclusive license to Springer Nature Switzerland AG 2025

This work is subject to copyright. All rights are solely and exclusively licensed by the Publisher, whether the whole or part of the material is concerned, specifically the rights of translation, reprinting, reuse of illustrations, recitation, broadcasting, reproduction on microfilms or in any other physical way, and transmission or information storage and retrieval, electronic adaptation, computer software, or by similar or dissimilar methodology now known or hereafter developed.
The use of general descriptive names, registered names, trademarks, service marks, etc. in this publication does not imply, even in the absence of a specific statement, that such names are exempt from the relevant protective laws and regulations and therefore free for general use.
The publisher, the authors and the editors are safe to assume that the advice and information in this book are believed to be true and accurate at the date of publication. Neither the publisher nor the authors or the editors give a warranty, expressed or implied, with respect to the material contained herein or for any errors or omissions that may have been made. The publisher remains neutral with regard to jurisdictional claims in published maps and institutional affiliations.

This Springer imprint is published by the registered company Springer Nature Switzerland AG
The registered company address is: Gewerbestrasse 11, 6330 Cham, Switzerland

If disposing of this product, please recycle the paper.

Contents

Achalasia

1

Ambre Nicolas, Melody Lopez, Miriam Sanz,
and Ana Martín-Nieto

1.1 Definition

Achalasia is a motor disorder of the esophagus characterized by the absence of peristalsis of the esophageal body and dysfunction of the lower esophageal sphincter (LES), which is unable to relax after swallowing. In other terms, achalasia is a rare distal motility disorder, in which the food bolus gets trapped in the sphincter, also known as the "cardias," on its way to the stomach and sometimes back up into the esophagus (Fig. 1.1) [1]. In this pathology, the neurons of the esophageal myenteric plexus are irreversibly destroyed [1].

1.2 Epidemiology

Epidemiological data indicate that in the United States and Europe, the annual incidence of this disease varies between 0.8% and 2% per 200,000 inhabitants [1]. In contrast, the annual incidence in places such as Africa appears to be significantly lower. Since achalasia is a chronic disease and its prevalence exceeds the incidence, it is estimated to be about 10 cases per 100,000 inhabitants. This condition can manifest itself at any stage of life, although it is most common between the ages of 30 and 60 years [1]. In terms of gender, it affects men and women almost equally. Despite cases of this disease have been documented in monozygotic twins and there is a certain familial aggregation, in most cases, there is no evident hereditary pattern [2].

A. Nicolas · M. Lopez · M. Sanz · A. Martín-Nieto (✉)
San Juan de Dios Foundation, Madrid, Spain

Department of Health Sciences, San Juan de Dios School of Nursing and Physical Therapy,
Comillas Pontifical University, Madrid, Spain
e-mail: amartinn@comillas.edu

© The Author(s), under exclusive license to Springer Nature
Switzerland AG 2025

J. Ruiz-Tovar, A. Martín-Nieto (eds.), *Physical Therapy for Gastrointestinal Disorders*, https://doi.org/10.1007/978-3-031-83651-0_1

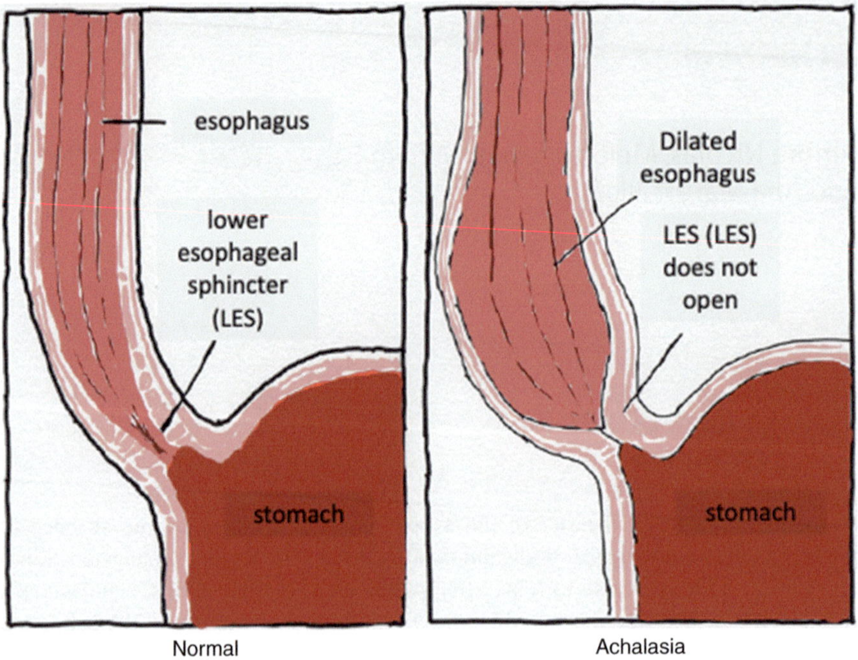

Fig. 1.1 Pathophysiology of achalasia

1.3 Etiology

The etiology of achalasia is unknown. The scientific literature indicates that the disease is secondary to a failure in the innervation of the smooth muscle of the esophagus [1].

Several theories try to explain the origin of the neurological disorder:

- Achalasia might be caused by a spontaneous degeneration of the neurons located in the spinal cord or in the myenteric plexus.
- Achalasia may be caused by a virus or other infectious agent.
- Recently, a hypothesis has emerged suggesting the existence of an autoimmune mechanism in achalasia. This theory is based on the observation of a significant association between this disease and human leukocyte antigen class II.

1.4 Pathophysiology

From a pathophysiological perspective, a set of changes occurring simultaneously is observed, leading to an imbalance in the normal functioning of the esophageal peristalsis. These abnormalities are due to the loss of myenteric plexus neurons [3]. As a result, there is a dysfunction in the relaxation of the LES, which should allow the proper passage of food into the stomach [4]. These abnormalities in the coordination and normal functioning of the esophagus can have significant implications on a subject's ability to effectively swallow and digest food [5].

1.5 Clinical Manifestations

This pathology may have a gradual onset with nonspecific symptoms, which may delay its diagnosis. The most common manifestation is dysphagia of solids that evolves to liquids and, subsequently, to regurgitation of soft foods or saliva. Other symptoms such as weight loss and chest pain may occur. This retrosternal pain improves with emesis of undigested food [2].

If the transit stops at the level of the cardias, food bolus accumulates in the body of the esophagus, leading to the appearance of symptoms such as:

- Need to cough to clear the throat after ingesting food and drink
- Coughing during or at the end of meals
- Fear at mealtimes
- Choking on certain foods
- Need to grind food to ingest it

1.6 Diagnostic Tests

A correct anamnesis is mandatory to know the main symptoms. Among the most relevant clinical manifestations are dysphagia for solids and liquids, regurgitation of undigested food, respiratory symptoms related with aspiration, chest pain, heartburn, and weight loss [6]. Complementary tests to confirm the diagnosis include [7]:

- *Upper digestive endoscopy:* the first step will always be to rule out an anatomical malformation or esophageal neoplasia. For this purpose, endoscopy is useful. This is an exploration of the esophagus, stomach, and duodenum through the mouth using an endoscope. The tube has a camera that allows the upper part of the digestive tract to be evaluated. Endoscopy can be normal in early stages of the disease. In advanced cases, endoscopy may reveal a dilated esophagus with retained food and a LES that remains continuously contracted and without the ability of relaxation. Mucosal erosions in the esophagus can be also observed as a result of the maintenance of the alimentary bolus during long time in the esophageal lumen.
- *Gastroduodenal esophageal barium swallow study:* It is a diagnostic procedure that uses x-rays to examine the esophagus. During this test, the patient swallows a liquid containing barium (contrast) that fills the lumen of the esophagus and allows the radiologist to clearly visualize its shape and function through a series of real-time x-ray images.

- *Esophageal manometry:* This procedure implies the insertion of a small pressure probe through the nose up to the stomach. Esophageal manometry allows to assess whether the esophagus is contracting and relaxing properly. Throughout the procedure, measurements will be taken of the pressure exerted by muscle contractions in different parts of the tube, including the LES and the body of the esophagus. Manometry evaluates the strength and progressiveness of the esophageal peristaltic wave and the relaxation of the LES to allow the emptying into the stomach. Typically, patients with achalasia showed vigorous contractions of the esophageal body and absence of relaxation of the LES.

1.7 Conventional Treatment

The two most used drugs are nitrates and calcium channel blockers. Nitrates inhibit normal LES contraction by dephosphorylation of the myosin light chain. Nifedipine, in sublingual doses of 10–20 mg 15–60 min before meals, is the most commonly used drug for achalasia. It inhibits LES muscle contraction by blocking cellular calcium uptake and reduces resting LES pressure by 30–60%. However, a major drawback of its use is the occurrence of side effects such as hypotension, headache, and dizziness in up to 30% of patients. In addition, tolerance to the drug develops over time [8, 9].

A widely used pharmacological treatment is topical injection of botulinum toxin type A, a neurotoxin that blocks the release of acetylcholine from nerve terminals. It is injected directly in a dose of 80–100 units in four or eight quadrants, into the LES through a sclerotherapy needle during upper gastrointestinal endoscopy. Botulinum toxin is a safe and effective treatment with few side effects [10]. The main drawbacks are that the effect of botulinum toxin is temporary, requiring new injections every 6–12 months, and the tolerance effect, requiring increasing doses of toxin in repeated procedures.

In addition to pharmacological treatment, other treatments options are discussed below.

1.7.1 Endoscopic Pneumatic Dilatation

Endoscopic pneumatic dilation is performed by inserting a balloon into the center of the LES during an endoscopy procedure, which is inflated to widen the opening. This procedure may need to be repeated on an outpatient basis if the esophageal sphincter does not stay open. Approximately one-third of people undergoing

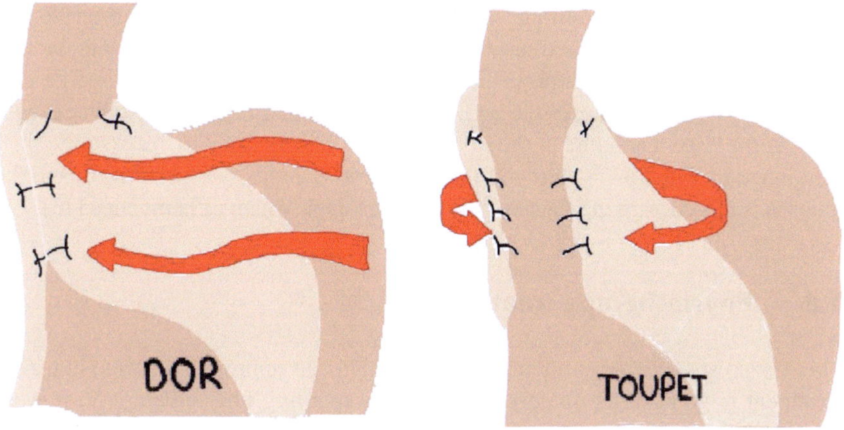

Anterior fundoplication
Posterior partial fundoplication

Fig. 1.2 Types of fundoplication

balloon dilation may need repeat treatment within 5 years. It is important to note that this procedure involves the use of sedation [12, 13]. This procedure also implies a significant risk of esophageal perforation.

1.7.2 Surgery: Heller Myotomy + Partial Fundoplication

This surgical procedure implies the division of the muscular layer (Heller myotomy) at the LES to avoid the concentrical contraction of the sphincter that closes the passage to the stomach. A sequelae of the myotomy is the loss of an anatomical anti-reflux system. To prevent further development of gastroesophageal reflux disease, a partial fundoplication is added to the procedure [11].

In fundoplication, the surgeon wraps the upper part of the stomach (fundus) around the lower esophagus to create an anti-reflux valve. This valve prevents acid from backing up into the esophagus, thus mitigating gastroesophageal reflux disease. Fundoplication can be performed on the anterior face of the esophagus (D'Or fundoplication) or on the posterior face (Toupet fundoplication) (Fig. 1.2) [11].

1.7.3 Peroral Endoscopic Myotomy

Peroral endoscopic myotomy (POEM) is a hybrid endoscopic surgical procedure that uses the concept of natural orifice transluminal endoscopic surgery to perform endoscopic myotomy. The POEM procedure involves the use of a high-definition overhead endoscope with a transparent cap attached to the tip. Using carbon dioxide insufflation and a specialized needle knife, an incision is made in the longitudinal mucosa in the lower esophagus proximal to the gastroesophageal junction. The submucosal space is then accessed, and a tunnel is created along the esophagus to a point in the lesser curvature of the stomach about 2–3 cm distal to the gastroesophageal junction. Finally, myotomy of the circular muscle fibers is performed, and the mucosa is closed with the linear and symmetric deployment of hemoclips [13].

1.8 Physiotherapy Treatment

There is no specific physiotherapy treatment that can improve achalasia; however, treatment is going to be mainly focused on respiratory physiotherapy to prevent complications, which could become seriously life-threatening for patients [14].

First, it will be necessary to perform an assessment of the patient. To evaluate its functionality, it will be necessary first to study the pulmonary volumes and capacities with a spirometer. Slow maneuvers should be performed to avoid the generation of irritative cough that could be annoying for the patient, either in sedentary, lateral decubitus, or prone/supine positions, reproducing the positions used throughout the day [14].

Then, the strength of the respiratory muscles (expiratory and inspiratory) will be evaluated with a pressure meter. Finally, the peak cough flow will be evaluated with a nasal gold mask connected to the spirometer. The maximum cough effort of the patient will be evaluated after a maximum pulmonary insufflation with an Ambu insufflator and with thoracic and abdominal pressures [14].

Physiotherapeutic treatment is adapted to each patient's situation and capacity, based on obtaining or maintaining good pulmonary/thoracic distensibility, facilitating the evacuation of secretions, removing them from the bronchial tree, improving swallowing, and providing education to patients and family members on techniques.

To improve dysphagia in patients, the following techniques can be used [14]:

- Active/resisted kinesitherapy of the tongue in various movements using the physiotherapist's finger to indicate directions. The strength and extension of the movement is worked.
- Stimulation of the swallowing reflex. Laryngeal mirror is introduced into the patient's mouth to touch the desired abutments and trigger the swallowing reflex.
- These exercises can also be combined with muscle electrostimulation for dysphagia by placing surface electrodes on the belly of the muscle to be stimulated (Fig. 1.3).

In the work of the thoracic part, techniques will be used to work on the patient's inspiration with an Ambu connected to a nasal mask, oronasal mask, or mouthpiece with a tube, allowing to synchronize the insufflation of air with the patient's inspiration. The aim is to reach maximum insufflation capacity, which means to reach the patient's maximum pulmonary capacity, with the assistance of the physiotherapist when necessary [7].

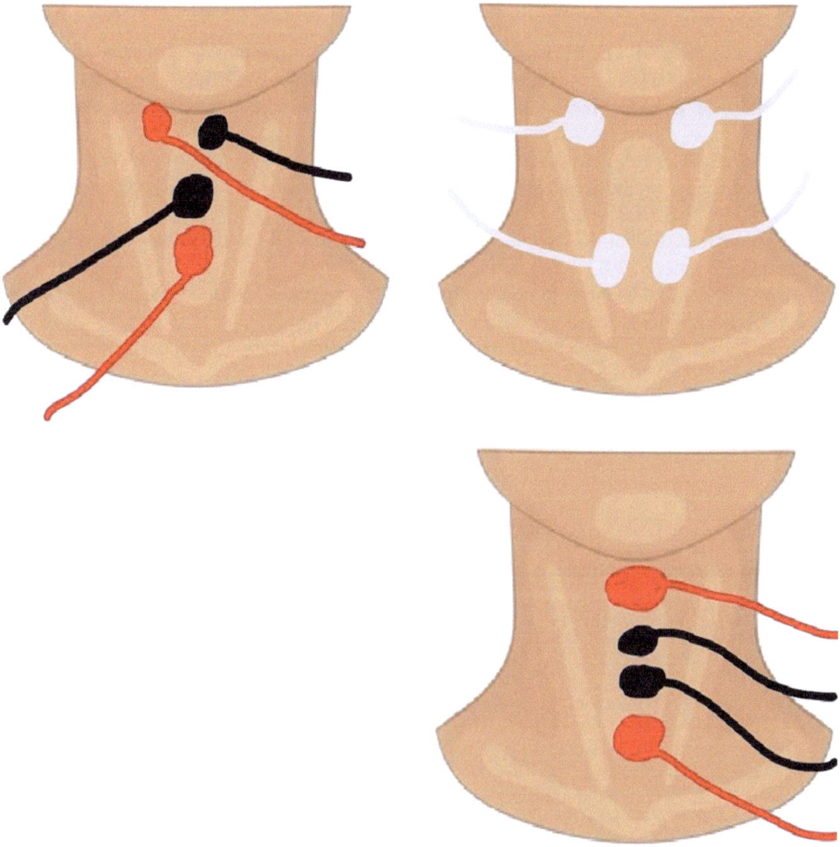

Fig. 1.3 Electrostimulation to treat dysphagia

References

1. Provenza CG, Romanelli JR. Achalasia: diagnosis and management. Surg Clin North Am. 2025;105(1):143–58.
2. Moonen A, Boeckxstaens G. Current diagnosis and management of achalasia. J Clin Gastroenterol. 2014;48(6):484–90.
3. Awaiz A, Yunus RM, Khan S, Memon B, Memon MA. Systematic review and meta-analysis of perioperative outcomes of peroral endoscopic myotomy (POEM) and laparoscopic heller myotomy (LHM) for achalasia. Surg Laparosc Endosc Percutan Tech. 2017;27(3):123–31.
4. Furuzawa-Carballeda J, Torres-Landa S, Valdovinos MÁ, Coss-Adame E, Martín Del Campo LA, Torres-Villalobos G. New insights into the pathophysiology of achalasia and implications for future treatment. World J Gastroenterol. 2016;22(35):7892–907.
5. Boeckxstaens GE. The lower oesophageal sphincter. Neurogastroenterol Motil. 2005;17(s1):13–21.
6. Gockel HR, Schumacher J, Gockel I, Lang H, Haaf T, Nöthen MM. Achalasia: will genetic studies provide insights? Hum Genet. 2010;128(4):353–64.

7. Hinkle JL, Cheever KH. Brunner & Suddarth's handbook of laboratory and diagnostic tests. Alphen aan den Rijn: Wolters Kluwer; 2017.
8. Gelfond M, Rozen P, Gilat T. Isosorbide dinitrate and nifedipine treatment of achalasia: a clinical, manometric and radionuclide evaluation. Gastroenterology. 1982;83(5):963–9.
9. Bortolotti M, Labò G. Clinical and manometric effects of nifedipine in patients with esophageal achalasia. Gastroenterology. 1981;80(1):39–44.
10. Leyden JE, Moss AC, MacMathuna P. Endoscopic pneumatic dilation versus botulinum toxin injection in the management of primary achalasia. Cochrane Database Syst Rev. 2014;2014(12):CD005046.
11. Kahrilas PJ, Pandolfino JE. Treatments for achalasia in 2017: how to choose among them. Curr Opin Gastroenterol. 2017;33(4):270.
12. Annese V, Bassotti G. Non-surgical treatment of esophageal achalasia. World J Gastroenterol. 2006;12(36):5763–6.
13. Arora Z, Thota PN, Sanaka MR. Achalasia: current therapeutic options. Ther Adv Chronic Dis. 2017;8(6–7):101–8.
14. Wilkinson JM, Codipilly DC, Wilfahrt RP. Dysphagia: evaluation and collaborative management. Am Fam Physician. 2021;103(2):97–106.

2 Functional Dyspepsia and Gastroesophageal Reflux Disease (GERD)

Álvaro Palomares, Joshua Cuariti, Ignacio Zambrano, and Ana Martín-Nieto

2.1 Definition

Functional dyspepsia and gastroesophageal reflux disease (GERD) are pathologies widely studied and reported in scientific literature, both related to gastrointestinal pathology.

Functional dyspepsia is related to chronic or recurrent upper abdominal pain located in the epigastrium [1]. Other studies define it as a series of medical symptoms that have their origin in the gastroduodenal region [2]. It should be noted that the terms defined are related only to "dyspepsia," but these same authors put the term "functional dyspepsia" in context by pointing out the origin of the pathology. Otero et al. [1] base their definition on the elaboration of an upper gastrointestinal endoscopy where no alterations are found to explain it. On the other hand, Meari [2] defines it as dyspepsia where there is no identifiable explanation for the symptoms, also called "non-organic dyspepsia," "idiopathic dyspepsia," or "essential dyspepsia."

The nomenclature GERD refers to gastroesophageal reflux disease. It can be defined as "that content that refluxes into the esophagus and generates bothersome symptoms and/or esophageal or extraesophageal complications." Furthermore, GERD refers to contents that reflux into not only the esophagus but also the oral cavity (including the larynx) and the lungs [3].

Á. Palomares · J. Cuariti · I. Zambrano · A. Martín-Nieto (✉)
San Juan de Dios Foundation, Madrid, Spain

Department of Health Sciences, San Juan de Dios School of Nursing and Physical Therapy, Comillas Pontifical University, Madrid, Spain
e-mail: amartinn@comillas.edu

© The Author(s), under exclusive license to Springer Nature Switzerland AG 2025
J. Ruiz-Tovar, A. Martín-Nieto (eds.), *Physical Therapy for Gastrointestinal Disorders*, https://doi.org/10.1007/978-3-031-83651-0_2

2.2 Epidemiology

Functional dyspepsia is a very common disease in the entire population. In North America, Europe, and Australia, the prevalence rate of functional dyspepsia is close to 50% [4]. Functional dyspepsia can appear at any age, although it mainly appears in the adulthood and is directly related to the lifestyle and diet of patients [4].

In relation to gastroesophageal reflux disease (GERD), a prevalence of between 10% and 20% can be identified in Europe and North America and 5% in the Asian continent [5]. Obesity is an important risk factor in the development of GERD; people with a high body mass index (BMI) are three times more likely to suffer this pathology than subjects with a normal BMI [6].

2.3 Etiology

Regarding functional dyspepsia, different risk factors have been established, such as female sex, infectious post-gastroenteritis state, diagnosis of anxiety disorder, and *Helicobacter pylori* infection [7].

Gastroesophageal reflux disease has a multifactorial origin. There are different causes that can provoke this pathology, such as an alteration in the anti-reflux barrier, anomalies in the lower esophageal sphincter (LES) or in the anatomic anti-reflux mechanisms, or a peristalsis that is not capable of mobilizing refluxed contents [8]. Some studies state that total or partial incompetence of the LES is the main cause of GERD [9]. On the other hand, the main mechanisms responsible for anti-reflux barrier dysfunction are LES hypotonia, inadequate transient relaxations of the LES, and hiatal hernia with dysfunction of the LES favoring gastroesophageal reflux [9].

2.4 Pathophysiology

The pathophysiology of functional dyspepsia is an evolving field that is not yet fully understood. It is believed to involve a complex interaction between several factors, including alterations in gastrointestinal motility, visceral hypersensitivity, abnormalities in sensory perception, and psychological disturbances [4]. Regarding gastrointestinal motility, irregularities in the contraction and relaxation of the muscles of the digestive tract have been observed, which may affect gastric emptying and lead to dyspepsia symptoms, such as early fullness and rapid satiety during meals [2]. Visceral hypersensitivity is another key aspect in the pathophysiology of functional dyspepsia. Patients with this disorder are thought to have an increased sensitivity to normal stimuli of the gastrointestinal tract, which may result in the perception of pain or discomfort even in the absence of structural or inflammatory abnormalities [10]. In addition, it has been shown that psychological factors, such as stress, anxiety, and depression, may play an important role in the development and exacerbation of symptoms of functional dyspepsia. These factors may influence the perception of pain and the response to gastrointestinal stimuli, which contributes to the complexity of the clinical picture of the disease [2].

GERD is a multifactorial condition involving the retrograde passage of acidic stomach contents into the esophagus, which can result in symptoms such as heartburn, acid regurgitation, and chest pain. The pathophysiology of GERD is related to several factors, including the function of the LES, esophageal and gastric motility, and the presence of hiatal hernia [9]. The LES plays a crucial role in the prevention of gastroesophageal reflux by acting as a physical barrier between the esophagus and the stomach. It has been shown that LES dysfunction, either by inappropriate relaxation or structural weakness, may predispose to the development of GERD. In addition, the presence of a hiatal hernia, which involves displacement of the stomach into the thorax through the esophageal hiatus, may contribute to reflux as it alters the anatomy and function of the LES [9].

2.5 Clinical Manifestations

Functional dyspepsia presents with a variety of symptoms that can significantly affect patients' quality of life. In addition to pain or discomfort in the upper abdomen, patients may experience a wide variety of symptoms, including early fullness, rapid satiety during meals, abdominal bloating, excessive belching, and nausea [2]. Importantly, symptoms of functional dyspepsia can be intermittent and vary in intensity, which can make diagnosis and management of the disease difficult. In addition, these symptoms may be chronic and recurrent, which can have a significant impact on the patient's quality of life, and require a comprehensive approach to disease management [10].

Symptoms of GERD can range from mild to severe and may include heartburn, acid regurgitation, chest pain, dysphagia, chronic cough, and hoarseness or sore throat. Importantly, symptoms of GERD may be intermittent and may be worse after meals, when lying down, or when leaning forward [9]. In addition, some patients may develop serious complications, such as erosive esophagitis, esophageal ulcers, esophageal stricture, or precancerous changes in the lining of the esophagus (Barrett's esophagus), which may require medical or surgical intervention [3].

2.6 Diagnostic Tests

The diagnosis of functional dyspepsia is based primarily on the exclusion of other organic causes of digestive symptoms. A thorough evaluation is required, which may include laboratory tests, such as blood tests, investigating for signs suggestive of infection or anemia, and imaging tests, such as abdominal ultrasound, CT scan, or upper digestive endoscopy, to rule out other gastrointestinal conditions [2]. In addition, specific tests to assess gastrointestinal function, such as esophageal manometry or esophageal pH-metry, may be performed to rule out motor or gastroesophageal reflux disorders. However, it is important to keep in mind that these studies may not be conclusive in the diagnosis of functional dyspepsia and should be interpreted in the patient's overall clinical context [9].

The diagnosis of GERD is based on clinical evaluation of the characteristic symptoms and can be confirmed by specific diagnostic tests. Endoscopy is useful to evaluate the esophageal lining and to rule out complications such as esophagitis or ulcers. Esophageal pH-metry is used to measure the amount and duration of acid in the esophagus, while esophageal manometry evaluates the function of the LES and esophageal motility [3].

2.7 Conventional Treatment

In the case of functional dyspepsia, there is not yet a treatment that is effective in all cases [2].

- *Diet:* dietary recommendations for functional dyspepsia include chewing properly and eating slowly. In addition, small, frequent meals should be eaten, and fat, tobacco, alcohol, and anti-inflammatory drugs should be avoided.
- *Drugs acting on gastric acid:* patients with functional dyspepsia are more sensitive to acid. Proton pump inhibitors (PPIs) reduce hydrochloric acid release. The antagonists of H2 receptors in the stomach also reduce acid secretion. These drugs are more useful in ulcerative-type functional dyspepsia.
- *Drugs that act on digestive motility:* these drugs are used when there is hypomotility of the stomach with slow gastric emptying, such as domperidone (a dopaminergic D2 antagonist) or cisapride (a serotonergic 5-HT agonist), but caution should be exercised with cisapride because of the adverse cardiac effects it can cause. The usefulness of prokinetics appears to be greater in dysmotility-type functional dyspepsia than in ulcer-type dyspepsia.
- *Drugs acting on visceral perception:* they decrease visceral hypersensitivity, such as drugs with hypoesthetic action. Fedotozin raises the threshold of perception and discomfort to intragastric distension. Synthetic somatostatin analogues (octreotide) can also be used with this aim.
- *Antidepressant drugs, anxiolytics, and psychotherapy:* selective serotonin reuptake inhibitors show a central analgesic effect as well as their antidepressant action. Anxiolytics are only indicated when there are associated psychofunctional alterations. Psychotherapy has been shown to be useful in certain cases.
- Eradication of *H. pylori*: its elimination produces benefits by improving chronic gastritis. In addition, it may decrease the risk of future peptic ulcers.

For the treatment of GERD, a number of measures may also be recommended, such as eating a healthy diet and avoiding fat-rich meals at least 2–3 h before bedtime [11, 12]. In addition, reducing body weight can help improve symptomatology, as this reduces the intra-abdominal pressure, which increases intragastric pressure and favors gastroesophageal reflux [13, 14]. With regard to pharmacological treatment, the following therapeutic options are recommended [15–19]:

- Antacids and alginates may be used for symptomatic relief.
- Histamine receptor (H2) antagonists can be used in cases of GERD with typical and sporadic symptoms.
- Proton pump inhibitors (PPIs) are the first choice for treatment. Although studies show variable rates of intragastric pH control and symptomatic response, meta-analyses have shown that effectiveness is similar among different PPIs [20].
- Prokinetics are used as a complementary treatment to PPI drugs, but never as the sole treatment.
- Inhibitors of transient relaxation of the LES (baclofen): There is moderate evidence that the use of the drug decreases transient sphincter relaxation, thus reducing reflux episodes (acid and non-acid). It is recommended as a complementary drug to PPIs.

Regarding surgical treatment, the current option is laparoscopic fundoplication [20].

2.8 Physiotherapy Treatment

A variety of physical therapy treatments have been explored to determine their efficacy in managing symptoms of functional dyspepsia. The following is a comprehensive overview of physical therapy treatments supported by current research:

- *Acupuncture:* the use of acupuncture has shown efficacy in the improvement of symptoms and quality of life in functional dyspepsia, even superior to the use of prokinetics [21].
- *Electro acupuncture:* there are different studies showing that treatment with electro acupuncture in patients with functional dyspepsia showed an improvement in dyspepsia symptoms by improving gastric pacemaker functionality and activity, neuropeptide Y levels, and gastrointestinal tract motility and enhancing vagus nerve activity [22, 23]. In addition, other studies share that transcutaneous electroacupuncture improves symptoms of functional dyspepsia, as well as quality of life, gastric regulation, and gastric emptying [24].
- *Transcutaneous electrical acustimulation:* may improve gastric accommodation and dyspeptic symptoms by increasing vagal activity and decreasing sympathovagal ratio [25].
- *Vacuum interferential current:* can improve epigastric discomfort, heartburn, bloating, early satiety, and postprandial satiety [26].

In the case of gastroesophageal reflux, respiratory exercise and manual therapy are recommended.

- *Myofascial relaxation:* a myofascial relaxation protocol performed on the diaphragm has shown an improvement in symptomatology and quality of life and a decrease in the use of PPIs [27].
- *Diaphragmatic breathing training:* the diaphragm is a key muscle in the prevention of gastroesophageal reflux. Diaphragmatic breathing exercises can strengthen the diaphragm, potentially improving its function and reducing GERD symptoms [28]. On the other hand, taking deep, slow breaths for 30 min every day, whether standing, sitting, or supine, produces an improvement in symptoms [28].
- *Respiratory muscle training:* Inspiratory muscle training focuses on strengthening the muscles involved in breathing, including the diaphragm, which can increase lower esophageal sphincter (LES) pressure and reduce reflux episodes [29].
- *Massage therapy:* Massage therapy aims to improve general well-being and reduce stress; thus, it can indirectly improve GERD symptoms [30].

Bibliography

1. Olson CG, Travers P, Lacy BE. Current opinion: functional dyspepsia. Curr Opin Gastroenterol (IF: 329; Q3). 2024;40(6):470–6.
2. Tran KT, Mai BH, Ta L, Dao LV, Tran HV, Tran MK, et al. Vietnam Association of Gastroenterology consensus for the diagnosis and treatment of functional dyspepsia. Clin Ter. 2024;175(5):307–17.
3. Shin A. Disorders of gastric motility. Lancet Gastroenterol Hepatol. 2024;9(11):1052–64.
4. Billey A, Saleem A, Zeeshan B, Dissanayake G, Zergaw MF, Elgendy M, Nassar ST. The bidirectional relationship between sleep disturbance and functional dyspepsia: a systematic review to understand mechanisms and implications on management. Cureus. 2024;16(8):e66098.
5. Veldman F, Hawinkels K, Keszthelyi D. Efficacy of vagus nerve stimulation in gastrointestinal disorders: a systematic review. Gastroenterol Rep (Oxf). 2025;13:goaf009.
6. Frieling T. Building a neurogastroenterology unit: why, where, and how? Visc Med. 2024;40(6):289–92.
7. Sarnelli G, Caenepeel P, Geypens B, Janssens J, Tack J. Symptoms associated with impaired gastric emptying of solids and liquids in functional dyspepsia. Am J Gastroenterol. 2003;98(4):783–8.
8. Sonu I, Oh SJ, Rao SSC. Capsules for the diagnosis and treatment of gastrointestinal motility disorders—a game changer. Curr Gastroenterol Rep. 2024;26(6):157–65.
9. Arín A, Iglesias MR. Enfermedad por reflujo gastroesofágico. Anal Sist Sanitari Navarra. 2003;26(2):251–68.
10. Chen H, He M, Cao J, Zhang Y, Zhou Y, Yu Q, et al. Acupuncture and moxibustion intervention in functional dyspepsia: gastric and duodenal regulation. Heliyon. 2024;10(17):e35696.
11. Duroux P, Bauerfeind P, Emde C, Koelz HR, Blum AL. Early dinner reduces nocturnal gastric acidity. Gut. 1989;30(8):1063–7.
12. Orr WC, Harnish MJ. Sleep-related gastro-oesophageal reflux: provocation with a late evening meal and treatment with acid suppression. Aliment Pharmacol Ther. 1998;12(10):1033–8.
13. Jacobson BC, Somers SC, Fuchs CS, Kelly CP, Camargo CA. Body-mass index and symptoms of gastroesophageal reflux in women. N Engl J Med. 2006;354(22):2340–8.
14. Katz PO, Gerson LB, Vela MF. Guidelines for the diagnosis and management of gastroesophageal reflux disease. Am J Gastroenterol. 2013;108(3):308–28.

15. Champion MC. Prokinetic therapy in gastroesophageal reflux disease. Can J Gastroenterol. 1997;11(Suppl B):55B–65B.
16. Ren LH, Chen WX, Qian LJ, Li S, Gu M, Shi RH. Addition of prokinetics to PPI therapy in gastroesophageal reflux disease: a meta-analysis. World J Gastroenterol. 2014;20(9):2412–9.
17. Vela MF, Tutuian R, Katz PO, Castell DO. Baclofen decreases acid and non-acid post-prandial gastro-oesophageal reflux measured by combined multichannel intraluminal impedance and pH. Aliment Pharmacol Ther. 2003;17(2):243–51.
18. Cange L, Johnsson E, Rydholm H, Lehmann A, Finizia C, Lundell L, et al. Baclofen-mediated gastro-oesophageal acid reflux control in patients with established reflux disease. Aliment Pharmacol Ther. 2002;16(5):869–73.
19. Gralnek IM, Dulai GS, Fennerty MB, Spiegel BMR. Esomeprazole versus other proton pump inhibitors in erosive esophagitis: a meta-analysis of randomized clinical trials. Clin Gastroenterol Hepatol. 2006;4(12):1452–8.
20. Gagné DJ, Dovec E, Urbandt JE. Laparoscopic revision of vertical banded gastroplasty to Roux-en-Y gastric bypass: outcomes of 105 patients. Surg Obes Relat Dis. 2011;7(4):493–9.
21. Zhang J, Liu Y, Huang X, Chen Y, Hu L, Lan K, et al. Efficacy comparison of different acupuncture treatments for functional dyspepsia: a systematic review with network meta-analysis. Evid Based Complement Alternat Med. 2020;2020:3872919.
22. Zheng H, Xu J, Sun X, Zeng F, Li Y, Wu X, et al. Electroacupuncture for patients with refractory functional dyspepsia: a randomized controlled trial. Neurogastroenterol Motil. 2018;30(7):e13316.
23. Liu S, Peng S, Hou X, Ke M, Chen JDZ. Transcutaneous electroacupuncture improves dyspeptic symptoms and increases high frequency heart rate variability in patients with functional dyspepsia. Neurogastroenterol Motil. 2008;20(11):1204–11.
24. Ji T, Li X, Lin L, Jiang L, Wang M, Zhou X, et al. An alternative to current therapies of functional dyspepsia: self-administrated transcutaneous electroacupuncture improves dyspeptic symptoms. Evid Based Complement Alternat Med. 2014;2014:832523.
25. Chen X, Chen X, Chen B, Du L, Wang Y, Huang Z, et al. Electroacupuncture enhances gastric accommodation via the autonomic and cytokine mechanisms in functional dyspepsia. Dig Dis Sci. 2023;68(1):98–105.
26. Köklü S, Köklü G, Ozgüçlü E, Kayani GU, Akbal E, Hasçelik Z. Clinical trial: interferential electric stimulation in functional dyspepsia patients—a prospective randomized study. Aliment Pharmacol Ther. 2010;31(9):961–8.
27. Zhang W, Shen Y, Hao J, Zhao Y. The role of psychotherapeutic approaches in treatment of functional dyspepsia, systematic review, and meta-analysis. Acta Gastroenterol Belg. 2024;87(2):294–303.
28. Zdrhova L, Bitnar P, Balihar K, Kolar P, Madle K, Martinek M, et al. Breathing exercises in gastroesophageal reflux disease: a systematic review. Dysphagia. 2023;38(2):609–21.
29. Casale M, Sabatino L, Moffa A, Capuano F, Luccarelli V, Vitali M, et al. Breathing training on lower esophageal sphincter as a complementary treatment of gastroesophageal reflux disease (GERD): a systematic review. Eur Rev Med Pharmacol Sci. 2016;20(21):4547–52.
30. Neu M, Pan Z, Workman R, Marcheggiani-Howard C, Furuta G, Laudenslager ML. Benefits of massage therapy for infants with symptoms of gastroesophageal reflux disease. Biol Res Nurs. 2014;16(4):387–97.

3 Gastritis and Gastroduodenal Ulcer

Tim Desgranges, Samuele Cugliari, Mathieu Grange, and Ana Martín-Nieto

3.1 Definition

Gastritis is a general term that can refer to an acute or chronic inflammation of the stomach lining caused by endogenous and exogenous factors that produces variable symptoms such as abdominal pain, nausea, and/or vomiting. If this gastritis is perpetuated over time, it can evolve into a gastroduodenal ulcer [1].

Gastroduodenal ulcers can be defined as excavated lesions on the mucosa that might affect the rest of the layers of the walls of the digestive tract, mainly in the stomach or in the duodenum [1].

Gastritis can be classified according to the severity and consequences of the inflammation into erosive gastritis and non-erosive gastritis.

Erosive gastritis is the most severe, due to its high inflammation and great wear and tear of the gastric mucosa. In comparison, non-erosive gastritis, as its name indicates, does not usually produce so much damage to the stomach mucosa. They can also be classified according to temporality into acute gastritis and chronic gastritis type A (chronic but very aggressive) and type B (persistent or recurrent). Acute gastritis is a self-limited alteration with regeneration and complete healing within a few days of eliminating the triggering agent. It appears suddenly, generally due to a bacterial infection, although it can be of viral or even fungal in origin in exceptional cases and, more specifically, due to the bacterium *Helicobacter pylori*, one of the few capable of resisting the acidity of the stomach. Chronic gastritis, however, has a prolonged duration, and its onset is not sudden. It begins with a mild or superficial

T. Desgranges · S. Cugliari · M. Grange · A. Martín-Nieto (✉)
San Juan de Dios Foundation, Madrid, Spain

Department of Health Sciences, San Juan de Dios School of Nursing and Physical Therapy, Comillas Pontifical University, Madrid, Spain
e-mail: amartinn@comillas.edu

© The Author(s), under exclusive license to Springer Nature Switzerland AG 2025

J. Ruiz-Tovar, A. Martín-Nieto (eds.), *Physical Therapy for Gastrointestinal Disorders*, https://doi.org/10.1007/978-3-031-83651-0_3

phase but progresses to a moderate stage (atrophic gastritis) and ends in gastric atrophy, by which time the stomach epithelium is almost completely destroyed [1].

Ulcers can be classified according to their location as duodenal ulcers, gastric ulcers, esophageal ulcers, or mouth ulcers. They can also be classified according to the mechanism of production into ulcers caused by stress, bacteria, or viruses [1].

3.2 Epidemiology

Gastritis has a significant morbidity worldwide and may affect 10% of the world's population at some point in their lives. It is also the most common cause of abdominal pain in the adult population [2].

Gastrointestinal ulcers, on the other hand, can appear at any age, being more frequent in adults between 40 and 65 years of age. In addition, between 50% and 70% of patients suffering from gastroduodenal ulcers present infection by *Helicobacter pylori* [3].

In terms of evolution and prognosis, patients with gastritis or gastrointestinal ulcers have very low mortality rates, thanks to pharmacological treatment. However, the probability of recurrence in the case of ulcers caused by *Helicobacter pylori* bacteria is very high, with a 50% risk of recurrence in the following 3 years. In addition, patients with ulcers have a 3–6 times higher risk of developing stomach cancer [4].

In general, both gastritis and ulcers may tend to become chronic. Their evolution depends, to a great extent, on the cause that provokes their appearance. In some cases, the etiology that triggers it can be treated, and the clinical manifestations disappear, although in other cases, the pharmacological treatment is aimed more at reducing the appearance of symptoms. However, it has actually a low mortality rate, with 2–3 deaths per 100,000 inhabitants, caused by the complications of ulcers [1].

3.3 Etiology

Infection by *Helicobacter pylori* bacteria is the most common cause of developing gastritis, but it can also be caused by other exogenous factors such as the use of nonsteroidal anti-inflammatory drugs (NSAIDs); gastric irritants such as drugs, alcohol, and tobacco; or exposure to radiation [5]. In addition, there are also endogenous factors that can provoke the appearance of gastritis such as gastric acid, pepsin, bile, pancreatic juice, urea, and some autoimmune disorders.

On the other hand, the main cause of the appearance of gastroduodenal ulcers is the bacterium *Helicobacter pylori* and the regular use of NSAIDs or other drugs such as corticoids or anticoagulants [1]. Other less common etiological factors are also described, such as intense physiological stress (which usually appear in burn patients, patients in critical condition, after major surgery, or with a cranioencephalic trauma). It can also appear in patients with some diseases such as Crohn's disease, Zollinger-Ellison syndrome, or infections caused by cytomegalovirus [6].

3.4 Pathophysiology

Gastritis can be defined as an inflammation of the gastric mucosa that occurs when there is an imbalance between cytotoxic and cytoprotective factors in the gastrointestinal tract. Depending on the degree of this imbalance, a more or less severe gastritis may develop, with variable consequences for the patient. Most abnormalities and imbalances are caused by the appearance of the bacterium *Helicobacter pylori*, which colonizes the gastric mucosa, damaging it to a variable extent. The presence of *Helicobacter pylori* produces a series of inflammatory mediators such as proteases, lipases, and cytotoxins [7].

Ulcers are described as erosive gastritis, caused by a rupture or ulceration in the protective mucosal lining of the esophagus. Peptic ulcers can be single or multiple, acute or chronic, and superficial or deep. Total ulcers extend through the muscular layer of the mucosa; damage the blood vessels, producing hemorrhage; or perforate the abdominal wall (Fig. 3.1). They may vary from millimeters to centimeters [7].

The causative factors, isolated or combined, produce an increased concentration of acid and pepsin (pepsin is produced by the principal cells of the gastric glands) that penetrate the mucosal barrier and lead to ulceration. The acid facilitates *Helicobacter pylori* infection. Perceived pain is the result of neurosensory stimulation by this acid [7].

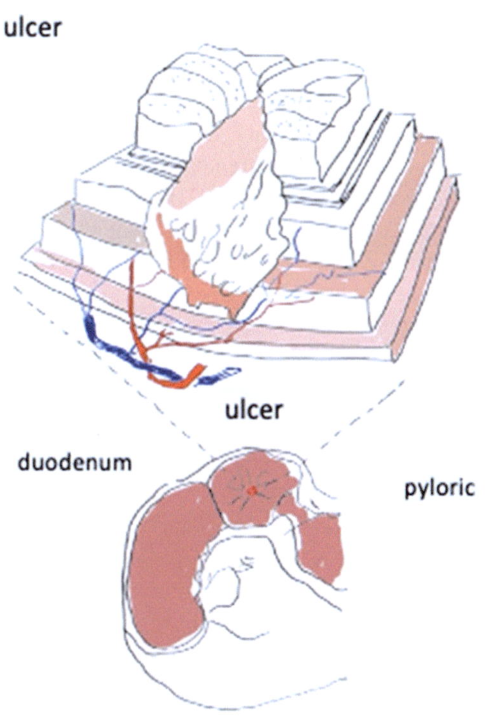

Fig. 3.1 Pathophysiology of gastrointestinal ulcers

3.5 Clinical Manifestations

The main clinical manifestations can be summarized in Table 3.1 [1, 6].

Complications of gastritis include the possibility of bleeding, development of gastric or duodenal ulcers, and gastric stenosis.

3.6 Diagnostic Tests

In most cases, it is necessary to perform a breath test or a stool test to rule out the presence of *Helicobacter pylori.* If pain and symptoms persist over time, an endoscopy can be performed to examine the gastric mucosa, to detect possible lesions and obtain biopsies. Upper endoscopy is a useful diagnostic test to confirm the presence of gastritis and to evaluate its severity mainly because of its ability to determine the underlying cause of the gastrointestinal symptoms. Endoscopic findings associated with these pathologies include edema, erythema, hemorrhagic mucosa, exudates, erosions, hyperplastic folds, and signs of mucosal atrophy [5].

Other laboratory tests may also be performed to determine whether antibodies to cytomegalovirus, herpes zoster, or syphilis or autoantibodies against gastric parietal cells are present [5].

3.7 Conventional Treatment

The pharmacological treatment used in gastritis and ulcers is aimed at reducing the acidity of the stomach. Among the drugs used are proton pump inhibitors, which aim to reduce and block acid production in the stomach for a prolonged period, thus promoting ulcer healing. H2 receptor antagonists, oral antacids, and gastric mucosal cytoprotectors can also be used [1]. In addition to pharmacological treatment, it will be necessary to carry out a series of general therapeutic measures to alleviate the symptomatology of the patients such as a diet free of irritating substances such as alcohol, tobacco, coffee, or spicy foods [1].

Table 3.1 Clinical manifestations of gastritis and gastrointestinal ulcers

Type	Clinical manifestation
Acute gastritis	Abdominal pain in the epigastrium, nausea and vomiting
Chronic gastritis	Sometimes, it is asymptomatic. If symptoms appear, they are similar to acute gastritis but persistent over time
Gastrointestinal ulcers	Epigastric abdominal pain described as corrosive and associated with nausea and vomiting. This pain begins 30 min to 2 h after ingestion; usually appears at night and decreases in the morning

3.8 Physiotherapy Treatment

There is currently no physical therapy treatment that significantly improves these pathologies. A recent study suggests that physical therapy may play an important role in the management of chronic gastritis by addressing and improving diaphragmatic and abdominal motility [8]. In addition, it has been shown that in subjects suffering from chronic gastritis, there may be an increase in musculoskeletal dysfunctions of the cervical spine with decreased rotation, lateral sliding, and pain on palpation [8]. By treating these consequences, as well as increasing diaphragmatic and abdominal mobility, there may be a partial improvement of the symptomatology.

Another study shows that physical activity can reduce the risk of gastrointestinal ulcers [9].

Finally, electro-acupuncture treatment has been experimented in rats; however, there is still no evidence to recommend its use in humans [10].

Bibliography

1. Valdivia RM. Gastritis y gastropatías. Rev Gastroenterol Peru. 2011;31(1):38–48.
2. Zuzek R, Potter M, Talley NJ, Agréus L, Andreasson A, Veits L, et al. Prevalence of histological gastritis in a community population and association with epigastric pain. Dig Dis Sci. 2024;69(2):528–37.
3. Feyisa ZT, Woldeamanuel BT. Prevalence and associated risk factors of gastritis among patients visiting Saint Paul Hospital Millennium Medical College, Addis Ababa, Ethiopia. PLoS One. 2021;16(2):e0246619.
4. Rappel S, Altendorf-Hofmann A, Stolte M. Prognosis of gastric carcinoid tumours. Digestion. 1995;56(6):455–62.
5. Goldenring JR, Mills JC. Cellular plasticity, reprogramming, and regeneration: metaplasia in the stomach and beyond. Gastroenterology. 2022;162(2):415–30.
6. Ramakrishnan K, Salinas RC. Peptic ulcer disease. Am Fam Physician. 2007;76(7):1005–12.
7. Lenti MV, Rugge M, Lahner E, Miceli E, Toh BH, Genta RM, et al. Autoimmune gastritis. Nat Rev Dis Prim. 2020;6(1):56.
8. Melo TM, Cunha FLL, Bezerra LMR, Salemi M, de Albuquerque VA, de Alencar GG, et al. Abdominal and diaphragmatic mobility in adults with chronic gastritis: a cross-sectional study. J Chiropr Med. 2023;22(1):11–9.
9. Cheng Y, Macera CA, Davis DR, Blair SN. Physical activity and peptic ulcers. Does physical activity reduce the risk of developing peptic ulcers? West J Med. 2000;173(2):101–7.
10. Xu J, Zheng X, Cheng KK, Chang X, Shen G, Liu M, et al. NMR-based metabolomics reveals alterations of electro-acupuncture stimulations on chronic atrophic gastritis rats. Sci Rep. 2017;7:45580.

Gastroparesis

4

Juan Sequí, Iván Simón, David Rubio, and Ana Martín-Nieto

4.1 Definition

Gastroparesis, also known as "delayed gastric emptying," is a pathology or chronic disorder based on the delay or arrest of the movement of ingested food from the stomach to the small intestine in the absence of mechanical obstruction of the gastric outlet. It is a gastric neuromuscular disease with motor and sensory dysfunction that causes chronic abdominal symptoms, limiting the quality of life of those who suffer from it [1].

4.2 Epidemiology

As for the epidemiology of this pathology, it may vary depending on many factors including the region or population studied [2]. The main data are summarized in Table 4.1.

4.3 Etiology

Gastroparesis can be explained by different causes, among which are the following [3]:

J. Sequí · I. Simón · D. Rubio · A. Martín-Nieto (✉)
San Juan de Dios Foundation, Madrid, Spain

Department of Health Sciences, San Juan de Dios School of Nursing and Physical Therapy, Comillas Pontifical University, Madrid, Spain
e-mail: amartinn@comillas.edu

© The Author(s), under exclusive license to Springer Nature Switzerland AG 2025
J. Ruiz-Tovar, A. Martín-Nieto (eds.), *Physical Therapy for Gastrointestinal Disorders*, https://doi.org/10.1007/978-3-031-83651-0_4

Table 4.1 Epidemiological data

Prevalence	It affects about 1–2% in developed countries, although it can increase up to 20% in certain populations such as people suffering from diabetes
Sex and age	It affects more women than men and usually young or middle-aged adults. It can also occur in children and older adults
Diabetes	It has been reported that 30–50% of people suffering from types 1 and 2 diabetes develop at least one episode of gastroparesis during their lifetime
Risk factors	Surgeries, disorders, and certain medications can be risk factors for this pathology
Bad habits	Tobacco and alcohol are not direct causes of the disease, but in some cases, they can lead to problems that trigger gastroparesis

Endocrine: by disorders in the release of hormones that affect food intake, such as satiety, or that produce inhibition of gastric emptying (such as cholecystokinin) and those that are responsible for the progression of the alimentary bolus in the digestive tract and its motility (insulin, GLP-1, etc.).

Infectious: in the case of certain bacteria and viruses, pathologies can develop in the digestive system that cause gastroparesis, such as gastroenteritis, although the infection can often arise from the accumulation of food in the stomach for a long time.

Neurological: affectations in the innervation responsible of intestinal and stomach motility and sensitivity, such as the vagus nerve, which is in charge of sending impulses through neurotransmitters to the smooth muscles of the stomach, can cause gastroparesis.

Metabolic: some conditions such as hypothyroidism, which slow metabolism, can affect gastric function, causing a decrease in bowel movements and increasing the risk of gastroparesis.

Idiopathic: when causes of gastroparesis are unknown.

Postoperative: after gastric surgery, gastric emptying may slow down. The section of the vagus nerve or some of their branches have been involved in the appearance of the disorder.

Ischemic: decreased blood flow to the stomach may result in slow gastric emptying.

Some common causes of this pathology are side effects of treatments such as chemotherapy or radiotherapy or even as a consequence of ingesting pain relievers, calcium channel blockers, or certain antidepressants [3].

4.4 Pathophysiology

Gastroparesis is a pathology associated with neuromuscular alterations in charge of gastric motility involving intrinsic enteric, extrinsic vagal, and motor innervation, since, either by an excess of esophageal motility or by relaxation of the esophageal sphincter, an excess of food can reach the stomach, producing an accumulation.

There may also be hypomotility of the smooth muscles of the stomach and intestine or contraction of the pyloric sphincter, which slows gastric emptying and the uptake of nutrients [1].

4.5 Clinical Manifestations

Clinical manifestations of gastroparesis are very heterogeneous, depending on the individual patient. In general, the most common manifestations are nausea and vomiting, as well as abdominal pain. In addition, other symptoms such as abdominal distention, heartburn, constipation, fever, early satiety, and postprandial fullness may also appear [1].

4.6 Diagnostic Tests

The diagnosis of gastroparesis should be made in patients presenting with symptomatology and demonstrating delayed gastric emptying, and other possible causes of gastric outlet obstruction have been excluded. Tests performed to obtain a diagnosis include:

Contrast-enhanced radiological techniques: this technique may suggest gastric retention due to deficient emptying of barium from the stomach, gastric dilatation, and presence of retained food. Lack of contrast emptying at 30 min and gastric retention at 6 h suggest gastroparesis. The major value of barium radiography is based on the exclusion of mucosal lesions and gastric mechanical obstruction [4].

Gastric emptying scintigraphy: it can be considered the ideal test for the diagnosis of gastroparesis. Solid emptying is a more sensitive indicator than liquid emptying, since liquid emptying may remain normal even in patients with advanced pathology [5]. It is preferable to perform the test 2–4 h after ingestion of food.

Breath test for gastroparesis: this is a test that measures gastric emptying using a non-radioactive carbon isotope that is administered together with a solid food and a short-chain triglyceride called octanate. After ingestion, substances are absorbed by the small intestine and metabolized into CO_2, whose measurement allows for the assessment of solid-phase gastric emptying [6].

Electrogastrography: this test is performed by placing skin electrodes on the abdominal wall to record gastric myoelectric muscle activity, which is responsible for controlling the maximum frequency and propagation of distal gastric contractions. The consumption of any food increases the amplitude of the electrogastrography signal, assuming an increase in antral contractility or mechanical distension of the stomach. The electrogastrography test quantifies the dominant frequency and regularity of gastric myoelectric activity, the percentage of time when abnormal slow wave rhythms exist during fasting and after ingestion, and assesses the increase in amplitude after a meal. An electrogastrography is considered abnormal when dysrhythmias occur for more than 30% of the recording time or when the consumption of a meal does not elicit an increase in signal amplitude [7].

Antroduodenal manometry: this is a test that evaluates gastric and duodenal motor function in both fasting and postprandial periods. It can be performed for short periods of 5–8 h but is usually performed on an outpatient basis for a period of 24 h, in which symptoms are correlated with abnormal motor patterns. It is especially indicated in patients with motor dysfunction with unexplained nausea and vomiting, patients with gastric or small bowel stasis, and patients with chronic intestinal pseudo-obstruction [8].

Ultrasound of the stomach: it allows the contour of the stomach to be examined. However, the efficacy of this test to evaluate the degree of gastric emptying depends on the experience of the operator, being only reliable to determine the rate of liquid emptying [9].

In addition to the aforementioned tests, MRI and proton emission tomography (PET) can also be used to evaluate gastric emptying [9].

4.7 Conventional Treatment

Patients suffering from gastroparesis must follow an adequate diet. In cases of mild gastroparesis, it will be sufficient if patients follow a series of guidelines including increasing nutrients in liquid form, since they are better digested; avoiding intakes that worsen distension, such as carbonated drinks; or gastric motility such as alcohol. In addition, it is preferable for patients to eat 4–5 small meals/day, where even homogenized or liquid meals supplemented with vitamins can be incorporated [10]. In most severe cases that do not respond to the above measures, jejunal feeding will be necessary. This procedure should be preceded by a trial of nasojejunal feeding for a few days, with infusion rates of at least 60 ml of iso-osmolar nutrient per hour. It is preferable to place jejunal feeding tubes directly into the jejunum, either endoscopically or laparoscopically, rather than through percutaneous endoscopic gastrostomy tubes. These probes make it possible to restore normal nutritional status, but are not free of adverse effects. It is important to allow a few days of habituation, gradually and slowly increasing the infusion rate from 10 ml/hour up to the target of 60 ml/hour [11]. As a last option, if the previous measures have not worked, parenteral nutrition should be prescribed, especially in cases of malnutrition. This should be a temporary measure to avoid the risk of infections and metabolic disturbances [11].

Pharmacological treatments include:

Metoclopramide: It is considered a first-line drug. It functions as a prokinetic because it has an antagonistic effect on the dopamine 2 receptor (D_2), promoting gastric emptying, and in addition, it binds to the 5-hydroxytryptamine 4 receptor

(5-HT4R) to stimulate cholinergic nerve pathways in the stomach [12]. Physiologically, it accelerates intestinal transit by increasing the tone and amplitude of gastric contractions, increases lower esophageal sphincter pressure, and improves antro-pyloro-duodenal coordination. In addition, this antiemetic agent provides relief through antagonism of central and peripheral dopamine receptors [13].

Domperidone: it exerts its prokinetic effect by being an antagonist of the D_2 receptors, thus improving the contractions of the antrum and duodenum and improving peristalsis. It also has antiemetic properties since it crosses the blood-brain barrier and acts on chemoreceptors located in the fourth ventricle [14].

Cisapride: cisapride promotes the release of acetylcholine in the myenteric plexus of the intestine and indirectly stimulates gastrointestinal motility. It acts as an agonist at 5-HT4 receptors and an antagonist at 5-HT3 receptors, both of which contribute to acetylcholine release and its subsequent prokinetic effects. Unlike metoclopramide, it lacks effects on the central nervous system due to its lack of antidopaminergic activity [15].

4.8 Physiotherapy Treatment

Gastric electrostimulation (GES) uses a small battery-powered device to deliver mild electrical impulses to the nerves and muscles in the lower stomach area. A surgical specialist implants this device under the skin in the lower abdominal region and connects the device's wires to the muscles of the gastric wall. Gastric electrostimulation can help reduce chronic nausea and vomiting. This procedure is used exclusively in the treatment of subjects suffering from gastroparesis associated with diabetes or of unknown etiology and only in patients whose symptoms do not respond to pharmacologic treatment. This technique is not exclusive to physiotherapy, although it can be used within physiotherapy in several ways [16].

In addition, physical activity performed during and after meals promotes evacuation of food from the stomach.

As a noninvasive treatment technique, transcutaneous electrical stimulation can be performed [17]. Transcutaneous peripheral nerve stimulation involves the application of electrical currents to the skin to stimulate specific nerves. Electrodes are placed on or near the nerves in the area to be treated. It is commonly used to treat chronic pain but has shown favorable results in the treatment of gastrointestinal disorders. The main techniques include transcutaneous vagus nerve stimulation (tVNS), transcutaneous sacral nerve stimulation (tSNS), and transcutaneous tibial nerve stimulation (tTNS).

Transcutaneous interferential current: interferential current dates back to the 1950s. IFC was initially used to treat genitourinary dysfunctions. Later studies found promising results in the treatment of gastrointestinal motility. The current is produced at the bisection of two diagonally opposite currents by their interference with each other. It generates a medium frequency current by using two sine waves that cross and interfere with each other, creating a third vector that penetrates nerve fibers deep in the target organs. A carrier frequency of 4–10 kHz has been used for two currents in IFC. However, 4 kHz was found to have better tolerability and optimal for penetrating deeper tissue.

Transcutaneous electrical acustimulation is a noninvasive, needle-free technique that applies electrical stimulation to the skin at acupuncture points via surface electrodes. This method evolved from traditional Chinese acupuncture or electroacupuncture, which involved needle puncture of an acupuncture point. It has been used to treat gastrointestinal disorders.

Bibliography

1. Zinsmeister AR, Szarka LA, Mullan B, Talley NJ. The incidence, prevalence, and outcomes of patients with gastroparesis in Olmsted County, Minnesota, from 1996 to 2006. Gastroenterology. 2009;136:1225–33.
2. Xv Y, Feng Y, Lin J. Efficacy and safety of acupuncture for postoperative gastroparesis syndrome: a systematic review and meta-analysis. Front Med (Lausanne). 2025;11:1494693.
3. Petrov RV, Bakhos CT, Abbas AE, Malik Z, Parkman HP. Endoscopic and surgical treatments for gastroparesis: what to do and whom to treat? Gastroenterol Clin N Am. 2020;49:539–56.
4. Parkman HP, Harris AD, Krevsky B, Urbain JL, Maurer AH, Fisher RS. Gastroduodenal motility and dysmotility: an update on techniques available for evaluation. Am J Gastroenterol. 1995;90(6):869–92.
5. Galil MA, Critchley M, Mackie CR. Isotope gastric emptying tests in clinical practice: expectation, outcome, and utility. Gut. 1993;34(7):916–9.
6. Bromer MQ, Kantor SB, Wagner DA, Knight LC, Maurer AH, Parkman HP. Simultaneous measurement of gastric emptying with a simple muffin meal using [13C]octanoate breath test and scintigraphy in normal subjects and patients with dyspeptic symptoms. Dig Dis Sci. 2002;47(7):1657–63.
7. Parkman HP, Hasler WL, Barnett JL, Eaker EY. American Motility Society Clinical GI Motility Testing Task Force. Electrogastrography: a document prepared by the gastric section of the American Motility Society Clinical GI Motility Testing Task Force. Neurogastroenterol Motil. 2003;15(2):89–102.
8. Barshop K, Staller K, Semler J, Kuo B. Duodenal rather than antral motility contractile parameters correlate with symptom severity in gastroparesis patients. Neurogastroenterol Motil. 2015;27(3):339–46.
9. Szarka LA, Camilleri M. Methods for measurement of gastric motility. Am J Physiol Gastrointest Liver Physiol. 2009;296(3):G461–75.
10. Camilleri M, Sanders KM. Gastroparesis. Gastroenterology. 2022;162(1):68–87.e1.
11. Limketkai BN, LeBrett W, Lin L, Shah ND. Nutritional approaches for gastroparesis. Lancet Gastroenterol Hepatol. 2020;5(11):1017–26.
12. Hoogerwerf WA, Pasricha PJ, Kalloo AN, Schuster MM. Pain: the overlooked symptom in gastroparesis. Am J Gastroenterol. 1999;94(4):1029–33.
13. Lata PF, Pigarelli DLW. Chronic metoclopramide therapy for diabetic gastroparesis. Ann Pharmacother. 2003;37(1):122–6.
14. Reddymasu SC, Soykan I, McCallum RW. Domperidone: review of pharmacology and clinical applications in gastroenterology. Am J Gastroenterol. 2007;102(9):2036–45.

15. Quigley EMM. Cisapride: what can we learn from the rise and fall of a prokinetic? J Dig Dis. 2011;12(3):147–56.
16. Parkman HP, Hasler WL, Fisher RS. American Gastroenterological Association technical review on the diagnosis and treatment of gastroparesis. Gastroenterology. 2004;127(5):1592–622.
17. Song G, Trujillo S, Fu Y, Shibi F, Chen J, Fass R. Transcutaneous electrical stimulation for gastrointestinal motility disorders. Neurogastroenterol Motil. 2023;35(11):e14618.

5 Chronic Nausea and Vomiting

Carlos Fernández-Calvo, Alonso Manuel García-Puga, José Luis Vicente-Arche, and Ana Martín-Nieto

5.1 Definition

Nausea is a subjective symptom and can be defined as an unpleasant sensation with an imminent need to vomit. Vomiting is a coordinated reflex of motor responses that results in the forced oral expulsion of gastrointestinal contents due to contraction of thoracic and abdominal wall muscles. When nausea and vomiting have a duration of more than 1 month, they are classified as chronic [1]. Vomiting should be differentiated from regurgitation and rumination. Regurgitation involves effortless and involuntary movement of gastric contents into the mouth without abdominal contraction [2]. It is a common symptom of gastroesophageal reflux. Rumination, however, can be defined as the effortless regurgitation of undigested food within minutes of starting or finishing a meal; the patient may swallow again or spit out the food [3].

According to Rome IV criteria [4], nausea and vomiting disorders include three subcategories: chronic nausea and vomiting syndrome, cyclic vomiting syndrome, and cannabinoid hyperemesis syndrome. The most common is chronic nausea and vomiting syndrome.

5.2 Epidemiology

In general, the epidemiology of chronic nausea and vomiting is still unknown. There are different studies and publications with different data depending on the causes and different populations. A study in the United States reported that 3.7% of

C. Fernández-Calvo · A. M. García-Puga · J. L. Vicente-Arche · A. Martín-Nieto (✉)
San Juan de Dios Foundation, Madrid, Spain

Department of Health Sciences, San Juan de Dios School of Nursing and Physical Therapy, Comillas Pontifical University, Madrid, Spain
e-mail: amartinn@comillas.edu

© The Author(s), under exclusive license to Springer Nature Switzerland AG 2025
J. Ruiz-Tovar, A. Martín-Nieto (eds.), *Physical Therapy for Gastrointestinal Disorders*, https://doi.org/10.1007/978-3-031-83651-0_5

emergency department visits were for nausea and vomiting. In the case of pregnant women, 56% of them present with vomiting during pregnancy [5]. Nausea and vomiting are also common in patients receiving chemotherapy; approximately 29% of patients undergoing chemotherapy may suffer from this symptomatology [6].

5.3 Etiology

There are various causes that can lead to the onset of nausea and vomiting. Among the most frequent causes is, as mentioned above, pregnancy. It is also frequent as an adverse effect of chemotherapy treatment (chemotherapy-induced nausea and vomiting). Table 5.1 summarizes different causes of nausea and vomiting [7].

5.4 Pathophysiology

Nausea and vomiting usually arise as a secondary symptom to other diseases, so they can occur for various reasons such as pregnancy or other pathologies, psychological disorders, or as an effect of any treatment (chemotherapy), among others. Another is when bacteria, viruses, fungi, toxins, and drugs enter the lumen of the gastrointestinal tract, they trigger a series of complex responses in the central nervous system, also causing vomiting [8]. The pathophysiological mechanisms involved have not been completely identified. The dorsolateral reticular formation of the spinal cord is known as the vomiting center. It is at this point that there is a convergence of the centers that coordinate the actions leading to vomiting (Fig. 5.1) [8].

Table 5.1 Etiology of nausea and vomiting

Anatomical causes	Gastric outlet obstruction, extraintestinal compression, pyloric stenosis
Hepatobiliary alterations	Acute and chronic hepatitis, biliary tract obstruction
Endocrine disorders	Diabetes mellitus, hyperglycemia, hyperthyroidism, Addison's disease, hypercalcemia
Vascular alterations	Superior mesenteric artery syndrome, chronic ischemia
Esophageal alterations	Achalasia, Zenker's diverticulum
Gastrointestinal disorders	Gastroenteritis, gastroparesis, adynamic ileus, non-ulcerative dyspepsia
Drugs and toxins	Antiarrhythmics, antibiotics, organophosphates, pesticides, arsenic, alcohol abuse, opioids, etc.
Psychiatric alterations	Anxiety and depression

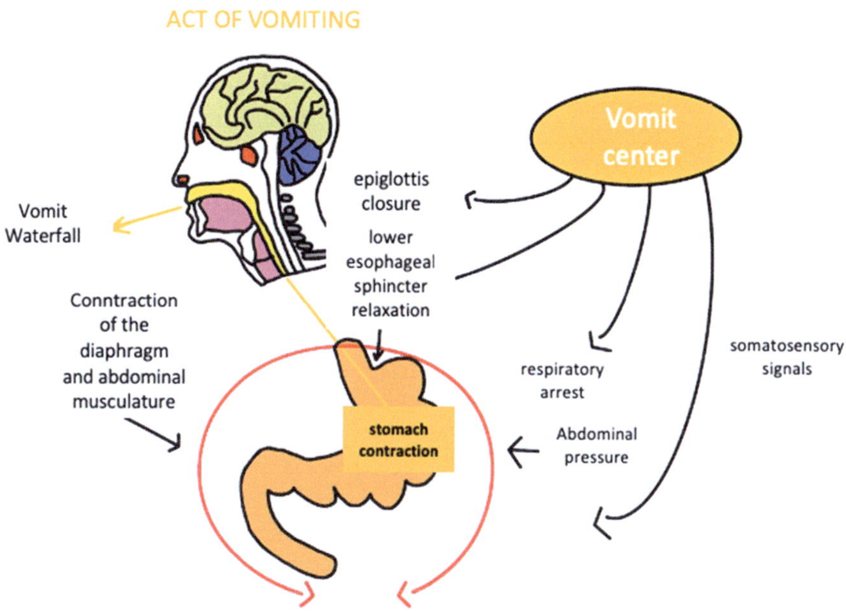

Fig. 5.1 Pathophysiology of vomiting

5.5 Clinical Manifestations

Chronic nausea and vomiting have several associated symptoms including abdominal pain, early satiety, and bloating. In addition, they may be accompanied by other symptoms to which special attention should be paid such as weight loss, anemia, or bleeding [7].

5.6 Diagnostic Tests

The aim of the diagnosis is to identify the cause of nausea and vomiting. In this case, it is essential to make a diagnosis through correct anamnesis and physical examination of the patient. Features of vomits often guide to the diagnosis: vomits with undigested food suggest a digestive disorder, hematemesis (vomits with blood) is frequent in neoplastic processes, and enteric or fecaloid vomits suggest a bowel obstruction. The performance of clinical tests should be guided by the clinical presentation, so a biochemical evaluation should be performed to determine hydroelectrolytic alterations or acid-base abnormalities up to the performance of specific diagnostic tests such as endoscopy to rule out other gastroduodenal diseases, intestinal obstruction, or cancer [2]. In addition, other imaging tests such as abdominal CT (computed tomography) may be performed to identify a possible intestinal obstruction. A scintigraphy may also be performed if gastroparesis is suspected. A contrast-enhanced gastrointestinal X-ray can rule out higher-grade proximal gastrointestinal lesions and obstruction. If GERD (gastroesophageal reflux disease) is suspected, pH measurement in the esophagus can be performed (pH-metry) [2]. Finally, serum tests can be performed to rule out hypothyroidism, Addison's disease, intoxication, or drug use. If all tests are negative, it may be diagnosed as chronic vomiting and nausea [2].

5.7 Conventional Treatment

Conventional treatment is mainly based on antiemetic drugs that help reduce nausea and the frequency of vomiting. Depending on the mechanism of action that causes vomiting, one type of drug or another may be used. Patients with chronic nausea and vomiting may benefit from liquid, dissolved, or parenteral presentations to maximize absorption and optimize pharmacokinetics. Table 5.2 summarizes the different drugs used [9].

In addition to pharmacological treatment, a series of measures and changes in habits can improve symptoms. In general, it is recommended to discontinue medications that decrease motility; in addition, it is important to have an adequate control of blood glucose levels and to follow a low-fat and low-fiber diet. On the other hand, it is necessary for patients to reduce consumption of alcohol and tobacco, since they can reduce intestinal transit [9].

In cases of continuous vomits despite antiemetic medication, bowel rest and insertion of a nasogastric tube can be indicated to empty the stomach, relieving the associated abdominal pain and nausea sensation. In such cases, correct intravenous hydration with hydroelectrolytic replenishment is mandatory, to prevent renal failure and even impairment of the nauseous and vomits.

5.8 Physiotherapy Treatment

Chronic nausea and vomiting can significantly affect patients' quality of life. Several physical therapy treatments have been explored to alleviate these symptoms. Below is a detailed description of the most relevant physical therapy interventions according to the most recent medical literature.

5.8.1 Gastric Electrical Stimulation (GES)

For the application of GES, a surgical procedure is necessary for the implantation of a device, which consists of two electrodes connected to a pulse generator. The electrodes are placed 1 cm and 10 cm from the pylorus, and the generator is placed sutured on the abdominal wall together with the battery, which lasts between 5 and 10 years. As for the parameterization, the standard configuration has been defined as pulse trains, with a train-on time set at 0.1 s and a train-off time of 5 s, a frequency of 14 Hz, a pulse width of 330 μs, and an amplitude of 5 mA [10, 11].

Table 5.2 Drugs used in chronic nausea and vomiting

Drug	Route of administration	Dose	Adverse effects
Antihistamine			
Meclizine	From 25 to 50 mg c/24 h	VO, IV	Dizziness, confusion, blurred vision, constipation, urinary retention
Diphenhydramine	From 25 to 50 mg c/6 to 8 h	OV, IV, IM	
Cinnarizine	From 25 to 75 mg c/8 h	VO	
Hydroxyzine	From 25 to 100 mg c/6 to 8 h	VO	
Phenothiazines			
Chlorpromazine	25–50 mg every 4–6 h	VO	Extrapyramidal reactions, neuroleptic malignant syndrome, QT interval prolongation
Perphenazine	From 4 to 8 mg c/8 h to 12 h From 5 to 10 mg/24 h	VO	
Thiethylperazine	6.5 mg c/8 h	VO, IV	
Dopamine receptor antagonists			
Metoclopramide	5–10 mg c/6 to 8 h	OV, IV, IM	Sedation, anxiety, dystonic reactions, extrapyramidal syndrome, galactorrhea, sexual dysfunction
Domperidone	10–20 mg c/8 h	VO	
5-HT4 receptor agonists			
Prucalopride	2 mg/d	VO	Headache and diarrhea
5-HT3 receptor antagonists			
Ondasetron	From 4 to 8 mg c/4 to 8 h	OV, IV, IM	Headache, discomfort, fatigue, constipation
Granisetron	1–2 mg c/12 to 24 h	VO, IV	
Neurokinin receptor antagonist			
Aprepitant	40–80 mg c/24 h	VO	Neutropenia, fatigue, headache, diarrhea, hiccups, constipation
Tricyclic antidepressants			
Amitriptyline	75–100 mg/day	VO	Constipation, agitation, sedation, delay of VG
Nortriptyline	10–25 mg/day	VO	
Neuromodulators			
Mirtazapine	15 mg/day	VO	Drowsiness, fatigue
Olanzapine	5–10 mg/day	VO	

OV oral route, *IV* intravenous route, *IM* intramuscular route, *GV* gastric emptying, *VG* gastric emptying

5.8.2 Spinal Cord Stimulation

Spinal cord stimulation seeks to reduce mainly abdominal and visceral pain; therefore, nausea and vomiting are reduced. A relationship has been demonstrated between conventional spinal cord stimulation and the enteric nervous system to alleviate visceral pain, nausea, and vomiting because sympathetic nerves carry nociceptive information from the viscera to the spinal nerve roots. To carry out this therapy, an implant is needed, as in the previous one, although this can be temporary or permanent. The parameterization of this treatment is as follows: electrodes are placed in the upper part of the vertebral bodies between T4 and T6, and frequencies of 40–90 Hz, pulse width of 240–400 ms, and amplitude of 3–8 mA are used [12].

5.8.3 Massage Therapy

A study demonstrated the benefits of massage in reducing nausea and vomiting in children after chemotherapy treatment. Swedish massage was performed with effleurage, petrissage, friction, and tapping movements with light-to-moderate pressure for 20 min [13].

5.8.4 Transcutaneous Electrical Stimulation of Acupuncture Points

Transcutaneous acupoint electrical stimulation (TAES) is a non-pharmacological method to prevent and treat nausea and vomiting. TAES can alleviate motion sickness, reduce the incidence of vomiting caused by chemotherapy, and treat pregnancy-induced nausea and vomiting. TAES has been shown to reduce the incidence of postoperative nausea after general anesthesia [14].

These physical therapy treatments offer several non-pharmacological options for managing chronic nausea and vomiting, providing significant symptom relief and improving patients' quality of life.

Bibliography

1. Hasler WL, Chey WD. Nausea and vomiting. Gastroenterology. 2003;125(6):1860–7.
2. Lacy BE, Weiser K, Chertoff J, Fass R, Pandolfino JE, Richter JE, et al. The diagnosis of gastroesophageal reflux disease. Am J Med. 2010;123(7):583–92.
3. Sasegbon A, Hasan SS, Disney BR, Vasant DH. Rumination syndrome: pathophysiology, diagnosis and practical management. Frontline Gastroenterol. 2022;13(5):440–6.
4. Sebastián Domingo JJ. The new Rome criteria (IV) of functional digestive disorders in clinical practice. Med Clin (Barc). 2017;148(10):464–8.
5. Getto L, Zeserson E, Breyer M. Vomiting, diarrhea, constipation, and gastroenteritis. Emerg Med Clin North Am. 2011;29(2):211–37, vii–viii.
6. Broder MS, Faria C, Powers A, Sunderji J, Cherepanov D. The impact of 5-HT3RA use on cost and utilization in patients with chemotherapy-induced nausea and vomiting: systematic review of the literature. Am Health Drug Benef. 2014;7(3):171–82.
7. Shin A. Disorders of gastric motility. Lancet Gastroenterol Hepatol. 2024;9(11):1052–64.

8. Zhong W, Shahbaz O, Teskey G, Beever A, Kachour N, Venketaraman V, et al. Mechanisms of nausea and vomiting: current knowledge and recent advances in intracellular emetic signaling systems. Int J Mol Sci. 2021;22(11):5797.
9. Kovacic K, Li BUK. Cyclic vomiting syndrome: a narrative review and guide to management. Headache. 2021;61(2):231–43.
10. Soliman H, Gourcerol G. Gastric electrical stimulation: role and clinical impact on chronic nausea and vomiting. Front Neurosci. 2022;16:909149.
11. Islam S, Vick LR, Runnels MJ, Gosche JR, Abell T. Gastric electrical stimulation for children with intractable nausea and gastroparesis. J Pediatr Surg. 2008;43(3):437–42.
12. Kapural L, Brown BK, Harandi S, Rejeski J, Koch K. Effects of spinal cord stimulation in patients with chronic nausea, vomiting, and refractory abdominal pain. Dig Dis Sci. 2022;67(2):598–605.
13. Mazlum S, Chaharsoughi NT, Banihashem A, Vashani HB. The effect of massage therapy on chemotherapy-induced nausea and vomiting in pediatric cancer. Iran J Nurs Midwifery Res. 2013;18(4):280–4.
14. Kramer BA, Kadar AG, Clark K. Transcutaneous acupoint electrical stimulation in preventing and treating nausea and vomiting in patients receiving electroconvulsive therapy. JECT. 2003;19(4):194.

Cholelithiasis

6

Pablo Meneses, Mateo Carbajo, Álvaro Escribano, and Ana Martín-Nieto

6.1 Definition

The presence of stones inside the gallbladder is called cholelithiasis. They can be composed of cholesterol (75%) or pigment stones formed by calcium salts of bilirubin. These stones appear in the gallbladder, but they can move into the biliary tract (<15%). It is an asymptomatic disease in most cases and is considered one of the most frequent pathologies of the gastrointestinal tract [1].

6.2 Epidemiology

Cholelithiasis is considered one of the most frequent pathologies of the digestive tract. Its incidence is affected by different factors such as ethnicity, sex, or age. It is more prevalent in women in developed countries, with a 2:1 ratio compared to men. This predisposition to appear in women may be due to a greater exposure to estrogens and progesterone. It is also related to age, being more prevalent in older people.

On the other hand, other factors such as a high-fat diet, obesity, and other hereditary diseases may increase the incidence [2]. In general terms, the worldwide incidence of cholelithiasis is between 10% and 30%, accounting for one million new cases each year [2].

P. Meneses · M. Carbajo · Á. Escribano · A. Martín-Nieto (✉)
San Juan de Dios Foundation, Madrid, Spain

Department of Health Sciences, San Juan de Dios School of Nursing and Physical Therapy, Comillas Pontifical University, Madrid, Spain
e-mail: amartinn@comillas.edu

© The Author(s), under exclusive license to Springer Nature Switzerland AG 2025

J. Ruiz-Tovar, A. Martín-Nieto (eds.), *Physical Therapy for Gastrointestinal Disorders*, https://doi.org/10.1007/978-3-031-83651-0_6

6.3 Etiology

There may be different predisposing factors, among which are the following [1]:

- Genetic factors: people with a family history of gallstones have a higher risk of suffering from this disease.
- Hormonal factors: possible hormonal variations in the body can become a trigger for gallstones and cholelithiasis to occur.
- Rapid weight loss: rapid weight loss leads to changes in bile composition, causing gallstones to occur.
- Obesity: Obesity is a factor that generates changes in the composition of bile and can produce gallstones. The risk is especially high in the case of morbidly obese women.
- Bile composition: high levels of cholesterol or bilirubin in the gallbladder may increase the likelihood of gallstones.

There may also be several protective factors such as:

- Moderate coffee consumption. The consumption of two or three cups of coffee can reduce the risk of suffering from symptomatic cholelithiasis by up to 40% [3].
- Consumption of vegetable protein [4].
- Consumption of monounsaturated and polyunsaturated fats in the context of a balanced diet may reduce the risk of cholelithiasis formation [5].
- Blood ascorbic acid levels above 27 μmol/l have a 13% lower risk of suffering cholelithiasis [6].

6.4 Pathophysiology

The pathophysiology of cholelithiasis formation can be defined on the basis of different phenomena described as follows [7]:

- Supersaturation of bile: bile is made up of different compounds such as cholesterol, bilirubin, and bile salts. When there is a change in the concentration of any of these components, bile can become saturated, thus favoring the formation of crystals.
- Nucleation: the cholesterol or bilirubin crystals that are present in the bile can stick together and cause solid nuclei to form, which are the initial gallstones.
- Growth and aggregation: gallstones can grow such that more crystals accumulate, and other components, such as proteins and inflammatory cells, are added.

Table 6.1 describes the different risk factors and their relationship to pathophysiology [7].

Table 6.1 Risk factors and pathophysiology

Age	Increased cholesterol secretion and decreased bile acid synthesis
Female gender	Increased cholesterol secretion and increased intestinal transit
Obesity	Hypersecretion of cholesterol into bile and increased cholesterol synthesis
Nutrition	Gallbladder hypomotility
Weight loss	Hypersecretion of cholesterol, decreased bile acid synthesis, and gallbladder hypomotility
Pregnancy	Hypersecretion of cholesterol, gallbladder hypomotility
Clofibrate	Increased cholesterol secretion
Contraceptives	Increased cholesterol secretion
Estrogens	Hypersecretion of cholesterol and decreased bile acid synthesis
Progestogens	Increased cholesterol secretion and hypomotility of the gallbladder
Octeotrid	Decreased gallbladder motility
Ceftriaxone	Precipitation in an insoluble salt of calcium-ceftriaxone
Genetic predisposition	Increased cholesterol secretion
Terminal ileum pathology	Hyposecretion of bile salts
Lower HDL	Increases HMG CoA reductase activity
Increased triglycerides	Increases HMG CoA reductase activity

6.5 Clinical Manifestations

In most cases, cholelithiasis is asymptomatic, when gallstones remain at the gallbladder without causing obstruction in the bile flow. However, when gallstones migrate from the gallbladder into the bile ducts, obstructing the normal flow of bile, this can cause symptoms such as biliary colic, acute cholecystitis, or pancreatitis.

The first symptoms that usually appear in patients are acute and recurrent abdominal pain known as biliary colic. This biliary colic is generally produced by a contraction of the gallbladder produced by hormonal and neural stimuli secondary to a partial obstruction of the cystic duct [8]. This pain is usually described as an intense oppressive pain in the right hypochondrium, in the epigastrium, or in the chest that radiates toward the back or the right scapular region [9]. In addition to this pain, other associated symptoms such as increased sweating, nausea, and vomiting may occur.

Choledocholithiasis appears when the lithiasis moves to the common bile duct. Its clinical presentation is usually abdominal pain on the right side due to spasm of the smooth muscle of the common bile duct, sometimes accompanied by jaundice and choluria. If the obstruction of the duct conditions a bacterial contamination, cholangitis (infection of the bile) can appear, which generally can cause bad general state, fever, and chills. Cholangitis is characterized by Charcot's triad, which is a set of three symptoms including fever, jaundice, and abdominal pain [10].

In several cases, the stones reach the Vater ampulla, which is the common end of the common bile duct and the Wirsung duct (pancreatic duct). In these cases, an obstruction in the release of pancreatic enzymes appears, which implies an inflammation of the pancreas [10].

Biliary ileus is a mechanical obstruction of the small bowel caused by the exit of a gallstone through a communication between the biliary tract and the intestine, the most frequent cause being cholecystoduodenal fistula [10]. Its typical clinical presentation is bloating and abdominal pain, vomiting, and absence of stool emission.

6.6 Diagnostic Tests

The test of choice for diagnosing cholelithiasis is usually abdominal ultrasound. This test stands out for being noninvasive and available to any health professional. Abdominal ultrasound is capable of detecting up to 98% of cases of cholelithiasis. In addition to abdominal ultrasound, it is important to carry out an adequate anamnesis and physical examination [11]. As for biochemical tests, in asymptomatic cholelithiasis, there are usually no significant alterations. In cases of biliary colic, liver enzymes (AST and ALT) are usually elevated. When an obstruction in the common bile duct is present, additionally, bilirubin or cholestasis enzyme (GGT and alkaline phosphatase) levels are increased. High concentrations of amylase and lipase in plasma are present in acute pancreatitis, reflecting the pancreatic cell damage with release of pancreatic enzymes [12].

Although abdominal ultrasound can be useful for the diagnosis of choledocholithiasis, magnetic resonance imaging is actually considered the gold standard. ERCP (endoscopic retrograde cholangiopancreatography) is also a useful tool for the diagnosis of choledocholithiasis. However, as it is an invasive procedure, actually, it is commonly used with therapeutic purposes [11, 13].

In biliary ileus, an abdominal X-ray can show dilated bowel loops, as a bowel obstruction. However, the cause of the obstruction cannot be evidenced as long as the calculus causing the ileum is not calcified. An abdominal CT (computed tomography) can be helpful to identify biliary ileus as the cause of the bowel obstruction, when pneumobilia (presence of air in the gallbladder) and ectopic gallstone are observed [12].

6.7 Conventional Treatment

First, patients diagnosed with cholelithiasis, especially when it is asymptomatic, should undertake a dietary change aimed at reducing fat content. In addition, they may benefit from a reduction in the consumption of foods such as milk and its derivatives, fatty sausages, eggs, and oil. The aims of these dietary changes are mostly focused on reducing the risk of becoming cholelithiasis symptomatic [14].

As for pharmacological treatment, there are specific drugs that can help improve lithiasis. Efficacy will depend on the size and composition of the stones. Patients with cholesterol-rich lithiasis without signs of calcification are candidates for treatment with bile acids and contact dissolution. If the lithiasis is larger, they may be candidates for lithotripsy combined with other techniques to favor dissolution of the stones [7].

One of the most commonly used drugs are bile acids, which act by inhibiting the formation of lithiasis and improving gallbladder emptying. The indication for the correct use of bile acids includes lithiasis smaller than 1 cm, mild symptoms, good gallbladder function, minimal calcification, and predominance of cholesterol in its composition. The most used acids are ursodeoxycholic acid and chenodeoxycholic acid. Ursodeoxycholic acid has fewer side effects, and its dose is 10 mg/kg. They have demonstrated their efficacy in reducing 90% of the stones formed. Despite its proven efficacy, stones dissolved by pharmacological treatment have a high incidence of recurrence, especially when there are multiple lithiasis and the time of disappearance has been slow [15]. Sometimes, HMG-CoA reductase inhibitors (statins) can be used. These agents reduce cholesterol secretion; however, they do not reduce cholesterol saturation.

Finally, extracorporeal lithotripsy can be performed through ultrasound. It is recommended in patients with less than three lithiasis, low body mass index (BMI), and good gallbladder function [7].

Although pharmacologic treatments can show a certain efficacy, surgical treatment with elective cholecystectomy is actually considered the gold-standard treatment for symptomatic cholelithiasis and in asymptomatic patients where the stones are >3 cm in diameter. The procedure is conducted by laparoscopic approach, which is associated with very low complications and mortality rates [7].

6.8 Physiotherapy Treatment

As for physiotherapy treatment, the following techniques can be used to improve symptomatology [14]:

- *Abdominal massage:* A massage would be performed in the abdominal area so that what we would get is better blood circulation, thus promoting better mobility also of the digestive system. This facilitates bile flow, reducing the risk of bile crystallization and gallstone formation.
- *Thermotherapy:* Heat therapy generates great benefits in terms of relieving the pain and discomfort of these gallstones, specially of the biliary colic. This would be applied to the abdominal region where the gallstones are located.

- *Regular physical exercise:* It is important to improve gastrointestinal function and to reduce possible symptoms that the patient may have, so we will ask the patient to do certain exercises.
- *Electrotherapy:* In this case, TENS would be used since, with a low-voltage current, the peripheral nerves are stimulated, thus relieving pain. The pain caused by gallstone complications is visceral pain. Visceral pain is carried by intercostal and abdominal wall nerves that conduct sensation from skin dermatomes and muscle fasciae. Electrotherapy can modulate the conduction of delta nerve fibers, mitigating pain.
- *Ultrasound:* It can be used to provide deep heat in the abdominal area, which relieves pain and reduces inflammation, as it helps blood circulation and aids in muscle relaxation.

References

1. Abdu SM, Assefa EM. Prevalence of gallstone disease in Africa: a systematic review and meta-analysis. BMJ Open Gastroenterol. 2025;12(1):e001441.
2. Park Y, Kim D, Lee JS, Kim YN, Jeong YK, Lee KG, et al. Association between diet and gallstones of cholesterol and pigment among patients with cholecystectomy: a case-control study in Korea. J Health Popul Nutr. 2017;36:39.
3. Leitzmann MF, Willett WC, Rimm EB, Stampfer MJ, Spiegelman D, Colditz GA, et al. A prospective study of coffee consumption and the risk of symptomatic gallstone disease in men. JAMA. 1999;281(22):2106–12.
4. Tsai CJ, Leitzmann MF, Willett WC, Giovannucci EL. Fruit and vegetable consumption and risk of cholecystectomy in women. Am J Med. 2006;119(9):760–7.
5. Tsai CJ, Leitzmann MF, Willett WC, Giovannucci EL. The effect of long-term intake of cis unsaturated fats on the risk for gallstone disease in men: a prospective cohort study. Ann Intern Med. 2004;141(7):514–22.
6. Simon JA, Hudes ES. Serum ascorbic acid and gallbladder disease prevalence among US adults: the Third National Health and Nutrition Examination Survey (NHANES III). Arch Intern Med. 2000;160(7):931–6.
7. Liepert AE, Ancheta M, Williamson E. Management of gallstone disease. Surg Clin North Am. 2024;104(6):1159–73.
8. Festi D, Sottili S, Colecchia A, Attili A, Mazzella G, Roda E, et al. Clinical manifestations of gallstone disease: evidence from the multicenter Italian study on cholelithiasis (MICOL). Hepatology. 1999;30(4):839–46.
9. Diehl AK, Sugarek NJ, Todd KH. Clinical evaluation for gallstone disease: usefulness of symptoms and signs in diagnosis. Am J Med. 1990;89(1):29–33.
10. Espinel J, Pinedo E. Choledocolithiasis. Rev Esp Enferm Dig. 2011;103(7):383.
11. Halabi WJ, Kang CY, Ketana N, Lafaro KJ, Nguyen VQ, Stamos MJ, et al. Surgery for gallstone ileus: a nationwide comparison of trends and outcomes. Ann Surg. 2014;259(2):329–35.
12. Vadher D, Zacken A, Shah V, Silmi M, Aguilar LS, Patel K, et al. The rolling stones: a systematic review and meta-analysis of the management of gallstone ileus. Chirurgia (Bucur). 2024;119(5):483–514.

13. Norero E, Norero B, Huete A, Pimentel F, Cruz F, Ibáñez L, et al. Accuracy of magnetic resonance cholangiopancreatography for the diagnosis of common bile duct stones. Rev Med Chile. 2008;136(5):600–5.
14. European Association for the Study of the Liver (EASL). EASL Clinical Practice Guidelines on the prevention, diagnosis and treatment of gallstones. J Hepatol. 2016;65(1):146–81.
15. Tomida S, Abei M, Yamaguchi T, Matsuzaki Y, Shoda J, Tanaka N, et al. Long-term ursodeoxycholic acid therapy is associated with reduced risk of biliary pain and acute cholecystitis in patients with gallbladder stones: a cohort analysis. Hepatology. 1999;30(1):6–13.

7 Meteorism and Belching

Lucas Molero, Sergio Gómez, Yago Iglesias, and Ana Martín-Nieto

7.1 Definition

Bloating is a very frequent abdominal symptom defined as a subjective sensation of excessive gas in the intestine that can manifest itself by bloating, excessive flatulence, abdominal pain, or even distension. It can be caused by different factors such as the consumption of certain foods or eating disorders. In general, it has a negative impact on the quality of life of those who suffer from it [1].

Among the main symptoms are abdominal discomfort and belching, the latter consisting of the expulsion of gas or air retained in the stomach, produced when food is ingested. Sometimes, it can be related to other digestive pathologies such as gastroesophageal reflux or gastritis [1].

7.2 Epidemiology

Meteorismus is a frequent gastrointestinal symptom whose epidemiology depends on different factors including diet, the presence of different digestive pathologies, or the state of the microbiota. In the general population, some studies suggest that it may occur at some time during the course of life in 48.8% of adults [2, 3]. In the case of children and adolescents, data can be found showing an incidence between 7% and 10% [4, 5].

L. Molero · S. Gómez · Y. Iglesias · A. Martín-Nieto (✉)
San Juan de Dios Foundation, Madrid, Spain

Department of Health Sciences, San Juan de Dios School of Nursing and Physical Therapy, Comillas Pontifical University, Madrid, Spain
e-mail: amartinn@comillas.edu

© The Author(s), under exclusive license to Springer Nature Switzerland AG 2025
J. Ruiz-Tovar, A. Martín-Nieto (eds.), *Physical Therapy for Gastrointestinal Disorders*, https://doi.org/10.1007/978-3-031-83651-0_7

7.3 Etiology

Meteorism, as a multisectoral phenomenon, refers to a clinical condition caused by an excess of gas in the intestine, provoked by different causes such as talking while eating, inadequate mastication and swallowing technique, smoking, or chewing gum. It is also often related to stress or the intake of foods rich in carbohydrates (non-absorbable fiber), sudden changes in diet, or taking antibiotics that alter the gut microbiota [6]. The gas contained in the intestine usually consists of N_2 (nitrogen), CO_2 (carbon dioxide), CH_4 (methane), and H_2 (hydrogen) and originates mainly from air ingestion and fermentation of certain foods, due to the intestinal microbiota [6].

As mentioned above, diet plays a fundamental role in the risk of suffering from meteorism. Table 7.1 summarizes the foods that produce a greater predisposition to meteorism.

It should be noted that there are other predisposing risk factors in addition to diet, such as underlying medical conditions such as digestive disorders, irritable bowel syndrome, or gastroesophageal reflux disease [6].

7.4 Pathophysiology

Meteorism usually occurs from the gastric cavity during or after eating. If the air travels caudally and reaches the stomach or upper parts of the intestine, it causes abdominal distention or pain, which tends to increase anxiety and continued swallowing of air.

Gas generation may also result from the fermentation of food in the stomach or in caudal regions of the small bowel or the colon [7]. This pathology may indicate the presence of gastrointestinal disorders such as [8]:

- Gastritis
- Gastroesophageal reflux, which causes regurgitation of gastric acid into the esophagus producing belching
- Irritable bowel syndrome, because it can affect the motility of the intestine and can contribute to gas retention and, to a certain extent, abdominal distention

Table 7.1 Food groups most likely to cause increased meteorism and belching

Food groups that are more likely to cause meteorism and belching	Examples
Cruciferous vegetables	Cauliflower, Brussels sprouts, cabbage, etc.
Legumes	Beans, lentils, and chickpeas
Foods rich in sorbitol	Apples, pears, plums, cherries, etc.
Dairy products	Especially to individuals who are lactose intolerant
Starch-rich foods	Potatoes, corn, and wheat

- Intolerance to certain foods
- Crohn's disease
- Bacterial overgrowth or dysbiosis

7.5 Clinical Manifestations

Among the clinical manifestations provoked by meteorism, the following can be highlighted [9]:

- Belching: release of air through the mouth.
- Abdominal distention: defined as a feeling of bloating or distension of the abdomen due to the accumulation of gas in the intestine.
- Flatulence: release of intestinal gas through the anus that may cause rumbling and odor.
- Abdominal discomfort: defined as pain or discomfort in the abdomen, which varies according to intensity.
- It can also cause a feeling of fullness that may be even after eating a small amount of food.

Patients frequently report that these symptoms increase and worsen throughout the day. These clinical manifestations affect the quality of life [9].

7.6 Diagnostic Tests

In most cases, the diagnosis is based mainly on anamnesis and physical examination. Occasionally, especially if the symptoms are severe or continuous, other diagnostic tests may be requested to rule out the presence of digestive diseases that may manifest themselves as meteorism [1]:

- Imaging tests: Contrast-enhanced gastrointestinal X-rays can be performed to rule out abdominal obstructions or gastric outlet difficulties that favor the fermentation of foods.
- Endoscopy: Upper digestive endoscopy and colonoscopy can be conducted when there is a suspicion of inflammatory bowel disease or neoplasms.
- Analysis of microbiota: The analysis of microbiota in the stools is increasingly performed to detect dysbiosis or bacterial overgrowth.

7.7 Conventional Treatment

In general, meteorism and belching do not require pharmacological treatment, and their intervention is usually aimed at changing certain habits or foods. Among the most common recommendations for these patients are the following [1, 10]:

- Avoid overeating. It is recommended to reduce food intake from 3 large meals to 4–7 small meals. This will help digest food better so that it does not produce gas in the intestine.
- Avoid foods rich in fats and carbohydrates, since they have a longer digestion and the symptoms of meteorism can be prolonged.
- Promote healthy eating patterns, including to avoid eating fast, so as not to ingest air in the process, and a correct mastication. Eating slowly helps better digest food, in addition to reducing the desire to continue eating.
- Avoid the intake of soft drinks during the meal or immediately after, since it can cause flatulence. Soft drinks, fruits, and vegetables should be consumed at least 1 h after the end of the meal.
- Avoid chewing gum, and do not drink through a straw.

There are some people who tend to suck in air when they get nervous. The best way to avoid this is to relax and reduce stress. Practicing breathing exercises in disciplines such as yoga and tai chi may be indicated in these cases [11].

In terms of food, it is recommended to avoid a long list of foods; among them are [11]:

- Lentils and beans, as they can generate gas when digested.
- Fruits and vegetables such as carrots, cauliflower, or Brussels sprouts.
- Foods with gluten.

In addition to change in eating habits, people prone to meteorism should be physically active, as this favors peristalsis and leads to expulsion of gases from the intestine.

As pharmacological treatment, medications may be used for the following purposes [1]:

- To relieve abdominal bloating by decreasing gas volume, such as those of the simeticone group (antiflatulents).
- To reduce pain or discomfort caused by gas (spasmolytics).
- Promote intestinal transit (prokinetics).

7.8 Physiotherapy Treatment

Physical therapy treatment for meteorism may vary depending on the cause and the patient's specific symptoms. Although physical therapy is not the primary approach to treating this pathology, there may be some techniques that can help alleviate symptoms.

Several studies have shown that moderate physical exercise can reduce intestinal gas accumulation and abdominal distention [12].

In addition, manual physiotherapy treatment may be performed to reduce symptomatology; among the treatments performed may include:

- Abdominal massage: gentle massage of the abdominal area can help stimulate movement and elimination of trapped gases in the intestine.
- Breathing exercises: some breathing techniques can help relax the abdominal muscles and promote gas release.
- Bowel mobilization exercises: specific exercises can help stimulate bowel movement and transit, which can help reduce gas accumulation.
- Electrical stimulation of dermatome T9: new research lines are actually focused on transcutaneous (TENS) or percutaneous (PENS) electrical neurostimulation of the periumbilical region (dermatome T9), whose preliminary results indicate that they promote peristalsis, reducing the time of fermentation of foods in the bowel and favoring the elimination of gas, finally leading to reduction of abdominal distension and symptomatic relief.

Bibliography

1. Crucillà S, Caldart F, Michelon M, Marasco G, Costantino A. Functional abdominal bloating and gut microbiota: an update. Microorganisms. 2024;12(8):1669.
2. Cockbain AJ, Parameswaran R, Watson DI, Bright T, Thompson SK. Flatulence after anti-reflux treatment (FAART) study. World J Surg. 2019;43(12):3065–73.
3. van Kerkhoven LAS, Eikendal T, Laheij RJF, van Oijen MGH, Jansen JBMJ. Gastrointestinal symptoms are still common in a general Western population. Neth J Med. 2008;66(1):18–22.
4. Devanarayana NM, Rajindrajith S. Aerophagia among Sri Lankan schoolchildren: epidemiological patterns and symptom characteristics. J Pediatr Gastroenterol Nutr. 2012;54(4):516–20.
5. Rana SV, Sharma S, Sinha SK, Kaur H, Sikander A, Singh K. Incidence of predominant methanogenic flora in irritable bowel syndrome patients and apparently healthy controls from North India. Dig Dis Sci. 2009;54(1):132–5.
6. Drossman DA. Functional gastrointestinal disorders: history, pathophysiology, clinical features, and Rome IV. Gastroenterology. 2016;150:1262–79.
7. Lacy BE, Cangemi D, Vazquez-Roque M. Management of chronic abdominal distension and bloating. Clin Gastroenterol Hepatol. 2021;19(2):219–231.e1.
8. Azpiroz F, Malagelada JR. The pathogenesis of bloating and visible distension in irritable bowel syndrome. Gastroenterol Clin N Am. 2005;34(2):257–69.
9. Floch MH. Netter, gastroenterology. Barcelona: Masson; 2006.
10. Harju E. The complaints and dietary habits of the patients with gastritis and undefined abdominal pain. Chir Ital. 1985;37(1):29–36.
11. Skuia NA, Burmeĭster MF, Zhikhar LI. Effect of a "green" diet on various clinical and metabolic indicators in patients with gastrointestinal diseases. Vopr Pitan. 1984;6:22–6.
12. Villoria A, Serra J, Azpiroz F, Malagelada JR. Physical activity and intestinal gas clearance in patients with bloating. Am J Gastroenterol. 2006;101(11):2552–7.

Inflammatory Bowel Diseases

8

Gonzalo García-Redondo, Raúl Chico-Barroso, Javier González-Martín, and Ana Martín-Nieto

8.1 Definition

Inflammatory bowel disease (IBD) comprises mainly ulcerative colitis, Crohn's disease, and indeterminate or unclassifiable colitis [1]. Crohn's disease can be defined as a chronic autoimmune inflammatory disease of the gastrointestinal tract with recurrent flares. The main symptoms include abdominal pain, diarrhea, fever, weight loss, and rectal bleeding. Crohn's disease can affect any part of the gastrointestinal tract, from the mouth to the anus. The most common location is the terminal ileum (the most distal part of the small intestine). It can also affect parts other than the digestive system, such as the joints, skin, liver, and eyes. It usually occurs in young people (between the ages of 20 and 30) but can occur at any age [2]. On the other hand, ulcerative colitis can be defined as a chronic inflammatory disease of the gastrointestinal tract that evolves periodically with flare-ups. Ulcerative colitis affects only the colon. It can also present manifestations outside the digestive system such as in the joints, skin, liver, eyes, etc. There is a greater probability of suffering from colon cancer after 10 years of having received the diagnosis of this disease [2].

8.2 Epidemiology

Regarding the epidemiology of inflammatory bowel diseases (IBD), an increase in incidence has now been observed in Europe and North America. Incidence varies by geographic area, ranging from 7 to 11 cases per 100,000 population in Europe and

G. García-Redondo · R. Chico-Barroso · J. González-Martín · A. Martín-Nieto (✉)
San Juan de Dios Foundation, Madrid, Spain

Department of Health Sciences, San Juan de Dios School of Nursing and Physical Therapy, Comillas Pontifical University, Madrid, Spain
e-mail: amartinn@comillas.edu

© The Author(s), under exclusive license to Springer Nature Switzerland AG 2025

J. Ruiz-Tovar, A. Martín-Nieto (eds.), *Physical Therapy for Gastrointestinal Disorders*, https://doi.org/10.1007/978-3-031-83651-0_8

the United States and 2–6 per 100,000 population in southern Europe, South Africa, and Australia. The lowest incidence rates are in Asia and South America [3]. About Crohn's disease, in recent years, an increase in cases has been observed in certain areas, reaching figures of 116 cases per 100,000 inhabitants [4].

Age and sex are other factors that influence the epidemiology of these diseases. Regarding age, there is a higher incidence between the second and fourth decade of life, with a higher mean age of presentation for ulcerative colitis than for Crohn's disease. Regarding gender, hardly any differences have been found between men and women.

8.3 Etiology

8.3.1 Crohn's Disease

Currently, Crohn's disease has an unknown cause; however, different investigations point to an increase of cases in genetically susceptible patients who present a bacterial or viral infection, supporting an autoimmune hypothesis. There are different risk factors that increase the risk of suffering from the disease [5, 6]:

- *Genetics and family history:* Studies refer to 71 genetic alterations, including those of the *NOD2/CARD* gene. Three alterations have been identified that are specifically related to Crohn's disease and to the alteration of the innate immune response, although they only occur in 10–30% of patients with Crohn's disease.
- *Environmental and dietary factors:* A diet rich in sucrose and carbohydrates, as well as high fat intake and decreased fiber intake, may increase the risk of Crohn's disease.
- *Infections:* Germs associated with increased risk of IBD include *E. coli*; *Yersinia enterocolitica*; *Clostridium*; *Campylobacte*r; *Wolinella*; *Mycoplasma*; *Chlamydia*; variants of *Pseudomonas*; *Mycobacterium paratuberculosis*, *avium*, and *kansasii*, *Simplexvirus*, and *Cytomegalovirus.*
- *Smoking:* In Crohn's disease, smoking can double the risk of developing the disease.

8.3.2 Ulcerative Colitis

Ulcerative colitis can be defined as a chronic inflammatory pathology, limited to the colon and rectum. It has an unknown etiology, although in genetically predisposed subjects, an exaggerated response of the immune system against the environment and the intestinal microbiota is suspected, causing inflammation and mucosal damage [7].

8.4 Pathophysiology

Crohn's disease begins with inflammation and abscesses of the crypts, which progress to small focal aphthoid ulcers. These mucosal lesions may progress to deep longitudinal and transverse ulcers with mucosal edema. Mesenteric fat usually extends over the serosal surface of the bowel. There is a demarcation between the pathologic bowel segments and the adjacent normal bowel, from which the name regional enteritis derives [8].

It is estimated that 35% of the cases of this disease involve only the ileum. Occasionally, the entire small bowel is affected. Involvement of the duodenum or esophagus is rarely seen, although there is often microscopic evidence of disease in the gastric antrum, especially in younger patients. In the absence of surgical intervention, the disease almost never spreads to regions of the small intestine unaffected at the time of initial diagnosis; after surgical resections, adjacent regions of the bowel can be de novo affected [8].

One of the complications that may appear is the increased risk of cancer in the affected small bowel segments. Patients with colonic involvement have an increased risk of colorectal cancer in the long term. Toxic megacolon may also be encountered, which is usually an uncommon complication of colonic Crohn's disease [8].

This disease can be classified into three main patterns, the first is mainly inflammatory that evolves over time, the second is stenotic or obstructive, and finally, the third is penetrating or fistulizing [8].

Ulcerative colitis in most cases usually starts in the rectum and remains there, causing ulcerative proctitis, but it often spreads upward, affecting the entire colon. The inflammation caused by this disease mainly affects the mucosa and submucosa, clearly limiting the normal and affected tissue. In the most severe cases, the disease involves the muscular layer of the mucosa, but penetration into deeper layers of the colonic wall, perforations, or fistulization is extremely uncommon. In the early stages, the mucosa is reddened, finely granular, and fragile, with loss of the normal vascular pattern, and often scattered hemorrhagic areas are observed. This disease reaches its highest level of severity when large mucosal ulcers with purulent exudate are produced. In contrast, no fistulas or abscesses are generated [9].

Table 8.1 lists the differences between the two pathologies.

Table 8.1 Differences between both pathologies

Crohn's disease	Ulcerative colitis
Erythematous/granulosa/edematous mucosa	Mucosa erythematous/granulosa/edematous
Aphthous, linear, and deep ulcers	Ulcers
Hemorrhages	Hemorrhages
Fistulas	Involvement of the rectum, sigma, and colon
Segmental nature of the lesion	Continuous inflammation

8.5 Clinical Manifestations

Crohn's disease manifests mainly with abdominal pain in the right lower abdomen, sometimes associated with other symptoms such as diarrhea, fatigue, weight loss, or fever. In addition to these digestive symptoms, it is often accompanied by various joint, skin, eye, or liver problems [10].

On the other hand, ulcerative colitis has gastrointestinal manifestations similar to Crohn's disease, but bloody diarrhea and rectal inflammation are more frequent [10].

8.6 Diagnostic Tests

The diagnosis of inflammatory bowel disease (IBD) is based on the integration of clinical, laboratory, endoscopic, and histological aspects.

To make the diagnosis, it is crucial to obtain a detailed clinical history that includes initial onset of symptoms, previous episodes, presence of rectal bleeding, frequency and characteristics of diarrhea, abdominal pain, changes in body weight, and the existence of perianal lesions. In addition, the presence of a family history of IBD, recent travel, use of anti-inflammatory medications, and history of infection should be assessed [11].

In addition to a detailed clinical history, biochemical, endoscopic, and imaging aspects must be taken into account for a diagnosis [11].

There is no specific test for IBD. The following clinical aspects and biomarkers will be taken into account to make a proper diagnosis:

1. Physical examination.
2. Laboratory tests: blood biometry, erythrocyte sedimentation rate (ESR), C-reactive protein, albumin, iron, ferritin, and stool examination (fecal calprotectin).
3. Elimination of the possibility of suffering from AIDS, tuberculosis, and other pathologies, such as intestinal infections, ischemia, etc.
4. Ileo-colonoscopy.
5. Abdominal ultrasound (US).
6. Magnetic resonance imaging (MRI) presents a higher diagnostic accuracy than computed tomography (CT).
7. Contrast-enhanced radiological examinations (intestinal transit and opaque enema) especially when MRI or CT is not possible.
8. Capsule endoscopy (when the previous ones have not been successful).

Despite advances in the identification of biomarkers for IBD, existing serological markers are insufficient for accurate diagnosis. Acute-phase reactants, such as CRP, lack specificity and should only be performed when IBD is suspected. In contrast, fecal markers, such as calprotectin, are more sensitive and specific for detecting intestinal inflammation and are therefore more widely recommended. Histological analysis is the only method to obtain a certain diagnosis.

8.6.1 Endoscopic Findings and Histopathological Analysis

When inflammatory bowel disease (IBD) is suspected, ileo-colonoscopy is considered the preferred method to confirm the diagnosis and evaluate the extent of the disease. In the specific case of Crohn's disease, one of its distinctive endoscopic features is the presence of inflammation distributed in irregular areas, with inflamed areas interspersed between normal-appearing mucosa. To diagnose both Crohn's disease and ulcerative colitis accurately, it is important to obtain biopsies from six different segments: terminal ileum, ascending, transverse, descending, sigmoid, and rectal. Ulcerative colitis typically shows a continuous affection of the entire colon (without normal-appearing mucosa sites) and sometimes extending to the terminal ileum, but the rest of the digestive tract remains unaffected.

It is important to note that histopathological diagnosis may be insufficient if biopsies are scarce, are not obtained from all the necessary segments, or are not well defined or, if clinical, endoscopic or histological parameters are missing to establish a clear diagnosis. When samples are sent for histological analysis, it is important to accompany them with the patient's clinical history, including age, duration, and type of disease, as well as details on treatment and endoscopic findings.

8.6.2 Imaging Tests

As for diagnostic imaging, different tests can be used:

1. Simple abdominal X-ray is usually used in patients with severe symptoms and serves to rule out intestinal obstruction. Specially in Crohn's disease, the appearance of bowel strictures in inflamed areas is typical, which may cause small bowel obstruction. In simple abdominal X-ray, usual findings of bowel obstruction can be observed, such as bowel loops dilation or bowel wall edema.
2. Intestinal transit with barium and barium enema. It is mainly used to assess small bowel involvement and can demonstrate thickened folds, stenotic segments with dilatation of proximal loops, fistulas, fissures, mucosal irregularity, rigidity, loop separation, cobblestone image, and abnormal peristalsis. The examination is contraindicated in uncontrolled ulcerative colitis in active phase.
3. Ultrasound. It can be used in the evaluation of transmural lesions in Crohn's disease when there is suspicion of abscess and in the diagnosis of hepatobiliary and nephro-urological complications.
4. Gammagraphy with marked leukocytes. It highlights areas of active inflammation. It has false negatives and positives.
5. Computed tomography and magnetic resonance imaging. They are useful for the evaluation of intestinal wall thickening, mesenteric fat alterations, and presence and size of lymph nodes. Pelvic MRI is an essential study in the evaluation of complex perianal disease.

8.7 Conventional Treatment

The treatment to address these diseases will depend on the severity of the condition and how the patient responds to the various medications used, following a stepwise approach. Topical treatments will be started, and then oral treatments will be considered, followed by rectal and, ultimately, intravenous treatments [12].

For mild IBD, it is recommended to initiate treatment with topical aminosalicylates. For induction of remission in patients with mild-to-moderate active idiopathic chronic ulcerative colitis with any extension beyond the rectum, treatment with oral aminosalicylates or sulfasalazine is recommended.

In addition, concurrent treatment with oral and topical aminosalicylates has been found to be more effective than oral aminosalicylates alone as first-line therapy for inducing remission in patients with mild-to-moderate active ulcerative colitis extending beyond the rectum [13].

In patients with moderate or severe IBD, oral systemic steroids are prescribed as the first option to induce clinical remission. In situations of acute severe UC requiring hospitalization, the use of intravenous systemic steroids, such as hydrocortisone or methylprednisolone, is suggested to induce remission [14].

To maintain remission in corticosteroid-dependent UC patients, the use of thiopurine immunosuppressants is recommended. Intravenous cyclosporine is recommended to be considered to induce remission in cases of severe active UC that do not respond to intravenous systemic steroids. In addition to these conventional approaches, there are treatments called biologics that are now widely used, although they are not considered within the category of conventional treatments. Biologic treatment consist in the administration of antibodies against specific targets of the inflamed cells. Immune-modulating drugs can also be used as adjuvant therapies, reducing the inflammatory response in the affected areas. In this line, metronidazole is widely used with an immune-modulating effect in cases of perianal affection in Crohn's disease [14].

Regarding surgical treatment, in ulcerative colitis, surgery is curative and should be resorted to in the case of severe flare-ups refractory to medical treatment or when it is not possible to achieve an adequate quality of life with medical treatment. Surgical treatment consists in total complete resection of the colon and rectum, with different options of reconstruction of the bowel transit. In the case of Crohn's disease, it is palliative and should be performed only for situations refractory to medical treatment and in selected cases, since there is a high rate of relapse [9]. In Crohn's disease, they are mostly indicated in cases of fistulas or strictures. As palliative procedures, it must be taken into consideration that eventual future new surgeries are possible. Thus, extensive surgical resections must be avoided, as future small bowel syndrome with severe nutritional consequences can be possible.

8.8 Physiotherapy Treatment

In addition to conventional medical and surgical treatment, physiotherapy treatment can be performed. The scientific literature recommends aerobic physical exercise for the improvement of symptoms in patients with Crohn's disease, as well as muscle-strengthening exercises [15]. In addition, due to the musculoskeletal consequences of both diseases, physical therapy can be applied to treat pain. Thus, kinesitherapy can be applied to mobilize the joints, stretching to stretch the musculature and relax it, and breathing exercises to work the diaphragm [15].

Physiotherapy is not only recommended as a treatment for musculoskeletal consequences of both diseases, but it is also indicated to work on the scar where abdominal surgery has been previously performed. The abdominal region is an area that is composed of different layers: the skin and subcutaneous cellular tissue, the superficial fascia, the deep fascia, the musculature that can vary depending on whether it is the anterior or lateral region, the extrapyramidal fascia, and the peritoneum. All these layers have to be crossed to access the digestive tract, so all of them are susceptible to poor scarring and irreversible adhesions. Physiotherapy can begin to work on the scar as soon as the stitches are removed, since the sooner it is started, the better the prognosis of achieving good healing. The techniques applied are deep and superficial transverse massages, fascial release techniques, dry needling, or diathermy [16].

Bibliography

1. Farrell D, McCarthy G, Savage E. Self-reported symptom burden in individuals with inflammatory bowel disease. J Crohns Colitis. 2016;10(3):315–22.
2. Floch MH. Netter, gastroenterology. Barcelona: Elsevier; 2006.
3. Borren NZ, van der Woude CJ, Ananthakrishnan AN. Fatigue in IBD: epidemiology, pathophysiology and management. Nat Rev Gastroenterol Hepatol. 2019;16(4):247–59.
4. Barberio B, Zamani M, Black CJ, Savarino EV, Ford AC. Prevalence of symptoms of anxiety and depression in patients with inflammatory bowel disease: a systematic review and meta-analysis. Lancet Gastroenterol Hepatol. 2021;6(5):359–70.
5. Fairbrass KM, Hamlin PJ, Gracie DJ, Ford AC. Natural history and impact of irritable bowel syndrome-type symptoms in inflammatory bowel disease during 6 years of longitudinal follow-up. Aliment Pharmacol Ther. 2022;56(8):1264–73.
6. Andoh A, Nishida A. Alteration of the gut microbiome in inflammatory bowel disease. Digestion. 2023;104(1):16–23.
7. Caruso R, Lo BC, Núñez G. Host-microbiota interactions in inflammatory bowel disease. Nat Rev Immunol. 2020;20(7):411–26.
8. Mills SC, von Roon AC, Tekkis PP, Orchard TR. Crohn's disease. BMJ Clin Evid. 2010;2010:0416.
9. Keshteli AH, Madsen KL, Dieleman LA. Diet in the pathogenesis and management of ulcerative colitis; a review of randomized controlled dietary interventions. Nutrients. 2019;11(7):1498.
10. Dinan TG, Cryan JF. Gut microbiota: a missing link in psychiatry. World Psychiatry. 2020;19(1):111–2.
11. Lind E, Fausa O, Elgjo K, Gjone E. Crohn's disease. Diagnostic procedures and problems. Scand J Gastroenterol. 1985;20(6):660–4.

12. Cottone M, Renna S, Orlando A, Mocciaro F. Medical management of Crohn's disease. Expert Opin Pharmacother. 2011;12(16):2505–25.
13. Schlussel AT, Cherng NB, Alavi K. Current trends and challenges in the postoperative medical management of Crohn's disease: a systematic review. Am J Surg. 2017;214(5):931–7.
14. Scherer M, Hardt J, Blozik E, Preiss JC, Bokemeyer B, Hüppe A, et al. Pharmacotherapy in patients with ulcerative colitis. Z Gastroenterol. 2011;49(7):820–6.
15. Pérez CA. Prescription of physical exercise in Crohn's disease. J Crohns Colitis. 2009;3(4):225–31.
16. Vavricka SR, Rogler G. Therapy of ulcerative colitis. Praxis (Bern 1994). 2009;98(4):209–12.

Diarrhea

9

Carlos Gómez, Lucia Carpintero, Marcela Marcial,
Alexandra Rivilla, and Jaime Ruiz-Tovar

9.1 Definition

The proper functioning of the digestive excretory system is essential for the organism as waste products are eliminated through defecation as a result of the digestion of food.

The small intestine and specially the colon are responsible for absorbing most of the water included in the alimentary bolus. The normal rhythm of defecation goes from three times a day to three times a week. If this rhythm is altered resulting in a volume greater than 250 g per day as well as stools of type 6 or 7 (lower consistency) according to the Bristol scale, it means that the water absorption mechanism is failing and resulting in diarrhea. Diarrhea may be accompanied by other symptoms such as fever, pain, or vomiting when it is caused by an infectious disease. However, there are cases of isolated diarrhea without accompanying symptoms [1, 2].

9.2 Epidemiology

The incidence will depend on specific factors such as hygiene practices, dietary habits, the geographic region, etc. The World Health Organization (WHO) estimates that 25% of the population suffers from at least one episode of acute diarrhea per year. 1.7 billion cases of diarrhea occur annually, and the majority of them are in tropical regions.

C. Gómez · L. Carpintero · M. Marcial · A. Rivilla · J. Ruiz-Tovar (✉)
San Juan de Dios Foundation, Madrid, Spain

Department of Health Sciences, San Juan de Dios School of Nursing and Physical Therapy, Comillas Pontifical University, Madrid, Spain

© The Author(s), under exclusive license to Springer Nature Switzerland AG 2025
J. Ruiz-Tovar, A. Martín-Nieto (eds.), *Physical Therapy for Gastrointestinal Disorders*, https://doi.org/10.1007/978-3-031-83651-0_9

The incidence recorded in relation to the adult population does not demonstrate definitive data due to the limited availability of data and ethological variants, due to the difficulty of studying feces of the different varieties of *E. coli*; however, it is estimated that the incidence of diarrhea in the adult population is 37.7–73.8% and varies depending on the definition applied.

There are studies that verify the impact of this clinical problem in hospitalized patients and how it can be a trigger for worsening for these patients and their treatment, becoming the most common non-hemorrhagic complication. In countries with better records, an estimate of 0.6 episodes per individual/year was found, figures from the United States and Germany.

There is more information and studies on the incidence in the pediatric population; an average of 7–30 episodes of diarrhea is reported in children under 5 years of age in developed countries, which is therefore one of the main causes of infant and child morbidity and mortality.

When children suffer several annual episodes of diarrhea, a collapse can occur at the circulatory level due to a lack of water and electrolytes, or it can affect the infection-malnutrition cycle, since it can cause nausea or vomiting, compromising growth and child development.

Acute infectious diarrhea is also a common cause of outpatient visits and hospital admissions in high-income regions and is a major health problem globally.

It is therefore an important cause of in-hospital involvement and therefore a clinical and epidemiological problem in pediatric units, especially in developed countries.

Most deaths from diarrhea are due to excessive fluid losses; these deaths are highly preventable [3].

9.3 Etiology

Diarrhea can be classified into different types according to its duration [4]:

- *Acute diarrhea.* Originated by various microorganisms such as viruses, parasites, bacteria, and fungi (Table 9.1) that cause infection; can be acquired in various ways by eating spoiled food and drinking contaminated water (Table 9.1).

Viruses and bacteria are the microorganisms that most frequently cause acute diarrhea because they are easily transmitted.

Table 9.1 Microorganisms causing acute diarrhea

Viruses	Parasites	Bacteria	Fungi
Norovirus	*Cryptosporidium*	*E. coli*	*C. albicans*
Adenovirus	*Giardia intestinalis*	*Salmonella*	*Aspergillus*
Rotavirus	*Entamoeba histolytica*	*Vibrio cholera*	

When a diarrhea is secondary to an infectious disease, it is commonly known as gastroenteritis. Its duration is usually less than 2 weeks, with spontaneous resolution within 48 h after contact with the microorganism in most cases. Although it is self-limiting, special care must be taken when this pathological process affects children, the elderly, and immunodeficient subjects, since the risk of severe dehydration and sepsis increases.

Microorganisms are not the only causes of acute diarrhea; other factors that might cause it are [4]:

- The intake of certain drugs, either because they contain some active ingredient that triggers it or because of the aggressiveness of the drug itself that comes to unbalance the intestinal flora.
- Psychosocial factors such as stress can cause diarrhea.
- Caused by other pathologies such as irritable bowel syndrome, fecal impaction, sepsis, etc.

- *Chronic diarrhea.* When diarrhea extends over time for more than 3–4 weeks, it is known as persistent diarrhea; if it does not subside in 4 weeks, we would be dealing with chronic diarrhea that in most cases occurs as a result of an intestinal disease such as in cancers affecting the digestive tract, endocrine tumors, or as a side effect of radiation treatment.

In addition to the duration, it is important to differentiate this pathological process according to its severity [1, 2]:

- Mild: It does not present with pain, and if there is pain, it is subtle. Daily bowel movements are 1–3 times, and since bowel movements are not numerous, it does not cause dehydration.
- Moderate: The number of bowel movements increases up to 5 times daily, pain is present, and fever does not exceed 38 °C. It still does not cause dehydration.
- Severe: It is described as producing more than five bowel movements per day. Pain is intense, fever reaches 40 °C, and dehydration begins.

9.4 Physiopathology

Knowing the causes is essential for the investigation of the origin that triggers this pathological process, to develop a better diagnosis and, therefore, a better treatment.

Diarrhea implies an increased secretion by all the cells and glands associated with the gastrointestinal tract, due to pathogens, toxins, or any other agent generating inflammation in the gastrointestinal tissues, provoking the liquid consistency of stools. In summary, one cause of watery diarrhea is the increase of liquid in the intestinal content [4].

The other cause of diarrhea involves the process of peristalsis, which is increased as an adaptive response of the organism in the presence of inflammation. The rapid peristalsis causes that the alimentary bolus to pass quickly from the stomach to the intestine and the colon, reducing the time for water absorption [1, 2].

Diarrhea can be also generated by an exudative cause, with alteration of the absorption function in the mucosa. The progressive destruction of the villi of the intestine can lead to diseases such as celiac disease or diseases affecting the gastrointestinal tract such as Crohn's disease or ulcerative colitis [1, 2].

9.5 Clinical Manifestations

The symptoms presented by the patient can also guide to the cause, especially when symptoms related to diarrhea are present:

- *Fever*. It is usually associated with the presence of invading pathogens. In childhood diarrhea, *Rotavirus* is almost always present.
- *Bloody stools*. These suggest the presence of invasive germs (*Salmonella*, *Campylobacter*, *Yersinia*, *Shigella*, *Amoeba*, invasive *E. coli*), cytotoxin producers (*Clostridium difficile*, enterohemorrhagic *E. coli*), or non-infectious diarrhea (ischemic colitis, ulcerative colitis).
- *Nausea and vomiting*. They are frequent in diarrhea of viral origin and those caused by bacterial toxins (e.g., *Staphylococcus aureus*). They are also frequent in cholera.
- *The occurrence of episodes of acid regurgitation*. Symptoms of reflux can be very varied: belching, epigastric pain, postprandial heaviness, nausea, hiccups, dysphagia, odynophagia (painful sensation when swallowing), pharyngeal and/or laryngeal discomfort, aphonia, respiratory disturbances, or chest pain. Some are not directly related only to diarrhea but also to other gastric pathologies.

9.6 Diagnostic Methods

Diagnostic must include anamnesis and physical examination, achieving a correct diagnosis in over 90% of cases with mild diarrhea.

In more severe situations, when signs of dehydration, toxicity, or dysentery diarrhea are present or in situations of higher risk, such as in the elderly, severely ill, or immunosuppressed patients and in those cases when it is not possible to establish the origin of the diarrhea, it may be necessary to perform complementary tests to confirm the etiology and select the proper treatment.

Complementary tests include:

- *Blood analysis*: It must include blood cell count and biochemical parameters, specially hydroelectrolytic ones (sodium, potassium, chloride, calcium, lactic acid, etc.), to rule out dehydration. Nutritional parameters (albumin, prealbumin,

retinol-binding protein, etc.) must also be assessed to evaluate the nutritional status, mostly in chronic diarrheas.
- *Stool analysis*: stool culture and antibiogram to identify a pathogen causing the diarrhea and the most adequate antibiotic treatment.
- *Abdominal imaging (X-ray plain films or CT scan)*: this can be useful for evaluating the presence of tumors, abdominal lumps, or partial intestinal occlusion.
- *Endoscopy*: Colonoscopy can be indicated in patients with bloody diarrhea and for differential diagnosis of organic causes (inflammatory bowel disease, radiation enteritis, etc.).

9.7 Conventional Treatment

The possibilities regarding the treatment of diarrhea are wide, and there is no definitive approach since the treatment will depend greatly on the etiology of the disease. The main objective of the treatment will be to improve the patient's symptomatology and try to mitigate the possible consequences of a prolonged diarrhea, such as dehydration, malnutrition, or dysbiosis [1, 5, 6].

- *Hydroelectrolytic Support*
- When oral intake is possible (in the absence of vomits), rehydration solutions must be administered to restore water-electrolyte balance. It aims to prevent dehydration caused by fluid loss in diarrhea, which may lead to acute renal failure. When oral administration is not possible, intravenous fluids must be prescribed [6].
- *Replenishment of Nutritional Deficiencies*
- In chronic diarrheas, it is common to find vitamin and mineral deficiencies. Thus, it is critical to replenish vitamins and nutrients lost due to lack of absorption. The route of delivery of these nutrients will depend on the patient's condition and the etiology of their illness [5, 6].
- *Dietary Modifications*
- Dietary modifications can positively alter the course of certain gastrointestinal conditions. For example, avoiding lactose- or gluten-containing foods can greatly benefit patients with lactose intolerance or celiac disease, respectively. Avoidance of lactose is also recommended in cases of extensive damage to the small intestine to decrease the delivery of large amounts of lactose and subsequent water retention in the colon.
- An astringent diet based on reducing the intake of foods moderately rich in fiber, fat, or lactose, among others, can be also beneficial [1, 5, 6].
- Additionally, the consumption of oral rehydration solution is important in cases of acute diarrhea.
- *Antibiotics*
- Diarrhea due to infectious agents is uncommon in developed countries. However, there is a population composed of travelers to tropical countries and immunocompromised patients that is considered a high risk. The main infectious agents

that usually cause diarrhea are *Clostridium difficile*, *Giardia lamblia*, and *Entamoeba histolytica*, among others. In these cases, treatment will be mainly based on the use of antibiotics. However, in developed countries, the main causes of infectious diarrheas are viruses; in such cases, antibiotics are not only useless but also harmful, as they might develop growth of multi-resistant bacteria and damage the intraluminal microbiota [1, 5, 6].

- *Absorbents*
- Absorbents act by binding to fluids, toxins, and other substances to improve stool consistency and eliminate toxins. Side effects include constipation and dark stools [1, 5, 6].
- *Probiotics*
- Probiotics are live microorganisms that can benefit the host. Their efficacy depends on the strain, dose, and viability of the microorganisms used in these preparations. The various mechanisms of action of probiotics include ability to adhere to the mucosa and compete with the pathogen for the mucosal adhesion, the ability to produce substances that act as a bactericide by breaking the pathogens, and the ability reproduce the pathogen itself unisexually to prevent it from attaching to the mucous layer [1, 5, 6].
- *Anticholinergics (Antispasmodics)*
- Anticholinergics are drugs that work through an effect on intestinal motility by blocking the binding of acetylcholine to its receptor. They reduce bowel motility and allow better absorption of water [1, 5].
- *Octreotide*
- Octreotide binds to somatostatin receptors found throughout the body and functions as an inhibitory hormone. The mechanisms of action of octreotide in the treatment of diarrhea include inhibition of the secretion of hormones such as gastrin, cholecystokinin, and secretin, which provoke increased water and electrolytic segregation by the gastrointestinal cells [1, 5].

9.8 Physical Therapy Treatment Options

The treatment of diarrhea can be a challenge that has been commonly oriented to pharmacological and dietary alternatives.

In recent years, the benefits of multidisciplinary management of chronic diarrhea have begun to be considered. Within the multidisciplinary team for the treatment of bowel dysfunctions, physiotherapy can play a key role, particularly from the perspective of manual therapy, as it has a great impact on the well-being of the tissues and the normalization of their function [7].

Visceral manual therapy has been found to have several positive effects such as the regulation of proinflammatory substances, psychological effect, and also an effect on pain relief. The latter is the most important for the physiotherapist as it can mean an improvement of the patient's clinical symptoms, thus improving their quality of life. In 2018, the physiotherapy school of Gimbernat University proposed a series of techniques and manual maneuvers for vagus nerve stimulation [8]. After analyzing the existing evidence, they concluded that the treatment of diarrhea from a physiotherapeutic approach should be based on the neuromodulation of this nerve since this could decrease intestinal permeability, increase tone, have anti-inflammatory action at the peripheral level, and modulate the composition of the microbiota, all beneficial effects for a patient with diarrhea. In the literature, we find a detailed description of techniques including nerve mobilization, jugular foramen decompression, mediastinal mobilization, and even manual therapy on the small intestine, large intestine, liver, gallbladder, and duodenum [8].

Following a similar line of research and in an attempt to expand the evidence relevant to this field of research, the University of Coruña conducted a systematic review of the application of manual therapy in bowel dysfunctions. They found that manual therapy has its main benefit on constipation and pain, bringing significant improvements in patients' symptoms and, as a consequence, quality of life. In this aspect, manual therapy could be used to treat symptomatology in a patient with diarrhea. However, the findings suggest that the treatment of diarrhea from a physiotherapeutic approach has little evidence [8].

As part of treatment, it is crucial to emphasize the importance of patient education toward independence. Emphasis should be placed on improving dietary habits and including exercise in lifestyle and stress management. Regular physical exercise can increase vagal tone, reduce inflammation, and even have a beneficial effect on stress, providing the patient with the necessary tools for self-management of the pathology. Stress, on the other hand, can cause inflammatory conditions, have a negative impact on the physiology of the intestinal tract, and even alter the composition of the microbiota. This aspect will be dealt with by a psychologist, but the physiotherapist can have an influence by identifying the events that most easily develop the patient's symptoms and by proposing a gradual exposure therapy to the event, that is, exposing the patient to the situation that causes anxiety and stress gradually in order to change the way the patient's body reacts to these events [8].

Bibliography

1. DuPont HL. Acute infectious diarrhea in immunocompetent adults. N Engl J Med. 2014;370(16):1532–40.
2. Sweetser S. Evaluating the patient with diarrhea: a case-based approach. Mayo Clin Proc. 2012;87(6):596–602.
3. Crockett ME, Keystone JS. Protection of travelers. In: Fischer M, Long SS, Prober CG, editors. Principles and practice of pediatric infectious diseases. Edinburgh: Elsevier Saunders; 2012. p. 82.
4. Wilson ME. Diarrhea in nontravelers: risk and etiology. Clin Infect Dis. 2005;41(Suppl 8):S541–6.
5. Li Z, Vaziri H. Treatment of chronic diarrhoea. Best Pract Res Clin Gastroenterol. 2012;26(5):677–87.
6. Grantham-McGregor SM, Walker SP, Chang S. Nutritional deficiencies and later behavioural development. Proc Nutr Soc. 2000;59(1):47–54.

7. Buffone F, Monacis D, Tarantino AG, Dal Farra F, Bergna A, Agosti M, Vismara L. Osteopathic treatment for gastrointestinal disorders in term and preterm infants: a systematic review and meta-analysis. Healthcare (Basel). 2022;10(8):1525.
8. Buffone F, Tarantino AG, Belloni F, Spadafora A, Bolzoni G, Bruini I, et al. Effectiveness of osteopathic manipulative treatment in adults with irritable bowel syndrome: a systematic review and meta-analysis. Healthcare (Basel). 2023;11(17):2442.

Irritable Bowel Syndrome

10

Arancha Ferrer, Elena Bueno, Ana Isabel Vegas, Inés Ca, and Jaime Ruiz-Tovar

10.1 Definition

Irritable bowel syndrome (IBS) is a chronic gastrointestinal disorder that affects the functioning of the large intestine. It is characterized by symptoms such as abdominal pain, changes in bowel habits (diarrhea, constipation, or alternating between both), abdominal distension, and general discomfort, which can vary in intensity and duration. Unlike other gastrointestinal diseases, IBS does not show specific structural abnormalities in conventional medical tests, being considered a functional disorder. Its exact causes are not fully understood, but it is believed to be related to visceral sensitivity, imbalances in intestinal microbiota, motility disturbances, and psychosocial factors. The diagnosis of IBS is based on excluding other conditions and the presence of characteristic symptoms. Treatment typically focuses on dietary changes, medications to control symptoms, and therapies for stress and anxiety management [1, 2].

10.2 Epidemiology

The literature studies the prevalence of IBS according to the diagnosis standards of Roma II. The IBS has an incidence of 10–20% in the general population, being the most common digestive illness in medical practices.

Gender affects disease epidemiology. For every man who suffers from IBS, there are two women. Gender also influences the subtype of IBS, having constipation and the alternation between diarrhea and constipation episodes in around 80% of IBS

A. Ferrer · E. Bueno · A. I. Vegas · I. Ca · J. Ruiz-Tovar (✉)
San Juan de Dios Foundation, Madrid, Spain

Department of Health Sciences, San Juan de Dios School of Nursing and Physical Therapy, Comillas Pontifical University, Madrid, Spain

© The Author(s), under exclusive license to Springer Nature Switzerland AG 2025

J. Ruiz-Tovar, A. Martín-Nieto (eds.), *Physical Therapy for Gastrointestinal Disorders*, https://doi.org/10.1007/978-3-031-83651-0_10

cases in women. In terms of symptoms, there are also some differences such as incomplete evacuation sensation, the presence of rectal mucus, or abdominal distension in women [1]. IBS is more common in individuals under 50 years, but it can also affect older adults as well [3]. However, some studies suggest that the probability of suffering from this illness decreases with age. Race appears to have no influence on IBS development.

IBS is often associated with other conditions such as fibromyalgia, chronic fatigue syndrome, gastroesophageal reflux disease (GERD), functional dyspepsia, and various psychiatric disorders including depression and anxiety. The symptomatology is sometimes so disabling that it is also a major cause of work absenteeism [1, 3].

10.3 Etiology

There are great knowledge gaps in the irritable bowel syndrome, but there are some aspects that have been involved with the disease [1, 3]:

- Abnormal muscular contractions in the intestinal walls: those that are stronger and longer lasting can cause gas, abdominal bloating, and diarrhea, while weaker contractions result in slower intestinal motility, leading to hard and dry stools.
- Nervous dyscoordination of signals between the brain and the bowel can lead to an exaggerated response to diverse stimuli during the digestive process, resulting in pain, diarrhea, or constipation.
- IBS sometimes appears following a severe viral or bacterial intestinal infection (gastroenteritis) or is associated with bacterial overgrowth in the intestinal flora or variations in the microbiota.
- Emotional factors such as stress, anxiety, or fear can trigger or worsen an irritable bowel syndrome flare-up. Individuals who experienced stressful events during childhood often have more symptoms of the disease in adulthood.
- Food allergies do not directly cause IBS symptoms, but for some patients, wheat, dairy products, legumes, caffeine, and certain fruits and vegetables can exacerbate the pathology. The high carbohydrate content of these foods leads to poor intestinal absorption and carbohydrate fermentation, resulting in gas cramps and abdominal bloating. High-calorie or high-fat diets also constitute a trigger for the onset of irritable bowel syndrome symptoms.
- Dysbiosis has been also associated with the development of the symptoms, frequently related with bacterial overgrowth.
- There is a certain familial aggregation, suggesting that there are probably genetic or hereditary factors involved.

10.4 Clinical Manifestations

Chronic functional digestive symptoms sometimes begin during the early childhood, including chronic diarrhea and functional abdominal pain.

In adulthood, symptoms are often of high intensity and can occur on more than 50% of days. However, there is a great interindividual variety in intensity and duration of the symptoms.

The main symptoms included in IBS are [1, 3]:

1. Abdominal pain and cramping: This is the most common symptom of IBS. The intensity can vary between different individuals and even in different moments for the same subject. It is usually relieved by defecation.
2. Altered bowel habits: IBS causes changes in bowel movements, including:
   - Diarrhea (IBS-D): frequent, loose, or watery stools.
   - Constipation (IBS-C): infrequent, hard, or lumpy stools.
   - Mixed (IBS-M): alternation between diarrhea and constipation episodes.
3. Bloating: bloating is also very frequent among IBS patients, and it can be uncomfortable and socially distressing.
4. Rectal tenesmus: incomplete evacuation is common.
5. Other symptoms associated with IBS include fatigue, sleep disturbances, anxiety, or depression.

The symptoms of IBS can be triggered or worsened by certain foods, stress, and hormonal changes [1, 3].

10.5 Diagnostic Methods

Diagnosing IBS involves a combination of medical history, symptom evaluation, and ruling out other conditions. Primarily, it must be taken into consideration that IBS is a diagnosis of exclusion, meaning that after ruling out other conditions, such as tumors or inflammatory bowel diseases among others, IBS is determined as the diagnosis [1].

Based on the findings, the most commonly diagnostic methods for IBS used are [4–6]:

- Rome IV Criteria: IBS is often diagnosed based on the Rome IV criteria, which include recurrent abdominal pain at least 1 day per week in the last 3 months, associated with changes in stool frequency and stool form (diarrhea or constipation).
- A scoring system based on patient history characteristics, physical examination, and basic laboratory investigations. The latter focus on erythrocyte sedimentation rate and blood count. This scoring system has been found to have good diagnostic accuracy, sensitivity, and specificity for IBS, making it a common diagnostic method.

- Additional blood tests to rule out conditions like celiac disease or infections. They must include complete blood count, biochemical and metabolic laboratory tests, as well as sedimentation rate and thyroid profile.
- Stoll test: to check for infections, inflammation, or malabsorption.
- Colonoscopy: recommended if there are suspicious symptoms of cancer or inflammatory bowel disease, like significant weight loss, anemia, a family history of colorectal cancer, or feces with pathological products like mucus, blood, or pus.
- Breath test: to check for bacterial overgrowth or lactose intolerance.
- Imaging tests: such as abdominal X-rays or CT scans to rule out other causes of symptoms.
- Another method focuses on short-chain fatty acids (SCFAs) in feces. These fatty acids have been recently evaluated as potential diagnostic biomarkers for IBS. The difference between levels of propionic and butyric acid in stool samples showed good diagnostic properties, with high sensitivity and specificity to distinguish between individuals with and without IBS. However, it is currently not used as a stand-alone diagnosis but as a supportive measure.

In conclusion, it is crucial to emphasize that these diagnostic methods should be used in combination with a comprehensive patient evaluation, patient history, physical examination, and exclusion of organic diseases to accurately diagnose IBS and avoid confusion with other intestinal conditions. The more precise the diagnosis, the more effective our treatment will be.

10.6 Conventional Treatment

The conventional treatment of IBS involves a combination of lifestyle changes, dietary changes, and medications to manage symptoms [1, 2].

1. Dietary changes:
   - Increasing fiber intake can reduce the symptoms, especially constipation. Fruits, vegetables, and whole grains are beneficial.
   - Foods that are high in certain fermentable carbohydrates, which can trigger symptoms, must be reduced or even avoided.
   - Other common triggers such as caffeine, alcohol, spicy foods, and certain artificial sweeteners must also be avoided.
2. Pharmacological drugs:
   - Antispasmodics can be useful to control abdominal pain.
   - Laxatives: for those with constipation.
   - Antidiarrheals: loperamide is commonly used to control diarrhea.
   - Antidepressants: they are also useful to relieve symptomatology, often associated with better control of anxiety or depression.
   - Probiotics: IBS has been sometimes associated with dysbiosis. Certain probiotics may balance gut bacteria.

3. Lifestyle modifications:
   - Techniques such as mindfulness, meditation, and yoga are helpful for stress management, which often exacerbates IBS symptoms.
   - Physical activity regulates bowel movements and reduces stress.
   - Cognitive behavioral therapy or hypnotherapy can be helpful to reduce stress and thereby relieve IBS symptoms.
4. Emerging treatments:
   - Fecal microbiota transplantation (FMT): This treatment involves transplanting stool from a healthy donor to restore healthy gut bacteria. This therapy has the same target as probiotics, balancing dysbiosis. However, FMT is still an investigational treatment, as it remains unclear for many pathologies what is a healthy donor.

10.7 Physical Therapy Treatment Options

The physiotherapeutic approach to treat IBS focuses on managing gastrointestinal symptoms and improving the patient's quality of life. While physiotherapy cannot cure IBS, it can provide relief and help control symptoms. Strategies used in this treatment include [7–9]:

- Manual therapy: involves gentle abdominal massages to reduce muscle tension and improve intestinal function.
- Therapeutic exercise: Involves specific exercises to strengthen abdominal muscles and promote a balanced intestinal motility, improving not only constipation but also diarrhea. Regular physical activity can also reduce stress, a common trigger for IBS. Various forms of exercise, including yoga, walking/aerobic physical activity, and tai chi, have been studied. Exercise significantly improved gastrointestinal symptoms, quality of life, depression, and anxiety.
- Biofeedback: Teaches patients to control muscle activity in the pelvic floor and intestinal area, improving intestinal function and reducing constipation or diarrhea symptoms. Rectal tenesmus can also show a significant relief[9].
- Relaxation and stress management techniques: physiotherapy may include deep breathing, guided visualization, and progressive muscle relaxation to reduce stress and anxiety, which can worsen IBS symptoms.
- Osteopathic manipulative treatment (OMT): visceral OMT reduces IBS symptoms and improves patient's quality of life.

It is essential to tailor physiotherapeutic treatment for IBS to each patient's individual needs. Collaboration with a multidisciplinary medical team, including physiotherapists, medical staff, and dietitians, is recommended to develop a comprehensive and effective treatment plan [7, 10].

Bibliography

1. Domingo JJ. Irritable bowel syndrome. Med Clín. 2022;158(2):76–81.
2. Tolliver BA, Herrera JL, DiPalma JA. Evaluation of patients who meet clinical criteria for irritable bowel syndrome. Am J Gastroenterol. 1994;89(2):176–8.
3. Marugán-Miguelsanz JM, Ontoria M, Velayos B, Torres-Hinojal MC, Redondo P, Fernández-Salazar L. Natural history of irritable bowel syndrome. Pediatr Int. 2013;55(2):204–7.
4. Chalubinski K, Brunner H. Positive diagnosis of irritable colon: a scored chart or standardized anamnesis? Wien Klin Wochenschr. 1987;99(23):819–24.
5. Kruis W, Thieme C, Weinzierl M, Schüssler P, Holl J, Paulus W. A diagnostic score for the irritable bowel syndrome. Its value in the exclusion of organic disease. Gastroenterology. 1984;87(1):1–7.
6. Farup PG, Rudi K, Hestad K. Faecal short-chain fatty acids—a diagnostic biomarker for irritable bowel syndrome? BMC Gastroenterol. 2016;16(1):51.
7. Coulis CM, et al. Physical therapy management for irritable bowel syndrome: a case series. J Women Health Phys Ther. 2015;39(3):128–35.
8. Brown A, et al. The role of physiotherapy in the management of patients with disorders of gut-brain interaction. J Neurogastroenterol Motil. 2019;25(2):205–10.
9. Lotfi C, Blair J, Jumrukovska A, Grubb M, Glidden E, Toldi J. Effectiveness of osteopathic manipulative treatment in treating symptoms of irritable bowel syndrome: a literature review. Cureus. 2023;15(7):e42393.
10. Varpio LE, et al. Pelvic floor physiotherapy for irritable bowel syndrome. Can J Gastroenterol. 2010;24(10):543–7.

11 Acute Diverticulitis

Álvaro Berdasco-Rodríguez, Diego Gil-Pastor,
Ana Gómez-Izquierdo, and Jaime Ruiz-Tovar

11.1 Introduction

Colonic diverticula are histologically pseudodiverticula or pulsion diverticula, as they are formed by herniation of the mucosa, muscularis mucosae, and submucosa of the colonic wall, but without affecting the muscular layers. These diverticula present as small protrusions in the colonic wall, formed by pressure exerted on weakened areas of the colonic wall [1].

Diverticular disease includes two forms of presentation [1, 2]:

- Diverticulosis: presence of colonic diverticula, which are often asymptomatic; when symptoms are associated, they are often mild.
- Acute diverticulitis: acute inflammatory condition of the colonic diverticula, mostly affecting the sigmoid colon. It can cause significant pain and discomfort in the lower abdominal quadrants. An inflamed diverticula is often accompanied by microperforations, allowing leakage of intestinal contents into the surrounding tissues or the peritoneal cavity, triggering local and systemic inflammatory response. Acute diverticulitis can be a life-threatening condition, and early diagnosis and adequate management are mandatory to avoid a fatal evolution.

Á. Berdasco-Rodríguez · D. Gil-Pastor · A. Gómez-Izquierdo · J. Ruiz-Tovar (✉)
San Juan de Dios Foundation, Madrid, Spain

Department of Health Sciences, San Juan de Dios School of Nursing and Physical Therapy, Comillas Pontifical University, Madrid, Spain

© The Author(s), under exclusive license to Springer Nature Switzerland AG 2025
J. Ruiz-Tovar, A. Martín-Nieto (eds.), *Physical Therapy for Gastrointestinal Disorders*, https://doi.org/10.1007/978-3-031-83651-0_11

11.2 Epidemiology

The prevalence of diverticular disease ranges between 20% and 60% in the general population. An increase of the prevalence is generally observed with the aging of the population, as diverticular disease is a degenerative disorder. Diverticular disease is the most frequent colonic pathology in the elderly, with a prevalence overcoming 65% in subjects over 80 years [1].

Diverticular disease is more frequent among females in the elderly, but a higher prevalence is observed among younger males [1].

There is a geographic influence of the disease. It is more common in Western and developed countries, where low-fiber diets contribute to its development [1, 2].

11.3 Etiology

Although a genetic predisposition has been described, showing familial aggregation, the most relevant factor leading to the development of diverticular disease is environmental ones. Lifestyle in developed countries, with a trend toward sedentarism and inadequate diets, leads to the development of diverticula and increases the risk of associated complications, mostly acute diverticulitis. A low intake of fiber (fruits, vegetables, cereals, legumes) provokes constipation, which has been closely related to diverticular disease. Sedentarism also induces a reduction of colonic peristalsis. Altogether, these factors increase the intraluminal colonic pressure and facilitate the herniation of pseudodiverticula in weakened locations of the colonic wall. In addition, obesity has been also associated not only with a higher prevalence of diverticulosis but also with an increased risk of acute diverticulitis [3].

Other factors associated with the appearance of diverticular disease include:

- Chronic intake of non-steroidal anti-inflammatory drugs (NSAIDs): These drugs reduce the synthesis of prostaglandins, which are essential components of the mucus barrier of the colon. The damage on the mucus barrier induces changes in the gut microbiota with an overgrowth of pathogen microorganisms involved in the inflammation of the diverticula.
- Opioids intake: they reduce colonic peristalsis and provoke constipation.
- Immune depression: The affection of the immune system facilitates inflammation and perforations of the diverticula. Complicated acute diverticulitis is more frequent among patients with immunological disorders.

11.4 Physiopathology of Acute Diverticulitis

Fecal material is introduced in the diverticula and inflames the mucosa and the diverticular wall. The progression of the inflammation can provoke a perforation of the wall and leakage of intraluminal colonic content (fecal material) into adjacent tissues of into the peritoneal cavity, provoking and acute peritonitis.

The severity of acute diverticulitis depends on the presence of perforations and the exit of fecal material into the peritoneal cavity [1–3].

11.5 Clinical Manifestations

Signs and symptoms of acute diverticulitis include severe abdominal pain, usually on the lower-left quadrant, fever, nausea, vomiting, and changes in bowel patterns, such as diarrhea or constipation. Abdominal tenderness and bloating are also common [1].

Complicated acute diverticulitis includes intra-abdominal abscess, fistula, and peritonitis. All these presentations are caused by a perforation. An intra-abdominal abscess is the consequence of a contained perforation, i.e., a small perforation in the diverticular wall is covered by the greater omentum, epiploic appendages, mesenteric fat, or even intestinal loops. The outflow of fecal material into the abdominal cavity is more limited and does not extend into the rest of the cavity. Clinically, it manifests as a mass within the abdomen [1, 3].

On the other hand, when the leakage of fecal contents extends throughout the peritoneal cavity, it is called acute peritonitis. Clinically, it appears as a picture of acute abdominal pain and shock, this being the most severe complication of acute diverticulitis. Peritonitis can be of fecal content or pus [1, 3].

Finally, diverticular perforation can communicate with neighboring hollow viscera and cause a fistula. The most frequent fistulas are with the bladder and in women with the vagina. Colovesical fistula manifests with pneumaturia, fecaluria, and repeated urinary tract infections, while colovaginal fistula is accompanied by leucorrhea, vaginitis, and leakage of feces through the vagina [1, 3].

11.6 Diagnostic Methods

Diagnosis of acute diverticulitis is made by imaging studies, such as abdominal CT scan, which may reveal inflammation, abscesses, or perforations. Colonoscopy, which is the diagnostic test of choice for diverticulosis, is contraindicated in acute diverticulitis, since the insufflation of air for the endoscopic procedure may cause perforation of an inflamed diverticulum [4].

11.7 Conventional Treatment

Treatment often involves the use of antibiotics to fight the infection, along with measures such as dietary changes, bowel rest, and analgesics.

In more severe cases, especially when there are complications such as extensive abscesses, fistulas, or perforations, surgical intervention may be necessary to remove the affected part of the colon. Adequate and timely management is crucial to prevent long-term or fatal complications.

The treatment of uncomplicated diverticulitis consists basically of antibiotics against anaerobic and gram-negative microorganisms. Classically, the antibiotic was administered intravenously associated with bowel rest, intravenous fluids, and pain control, all of them requiring hospital admission. However, nowadays, the possibility of outpatient treatment is contemplated in milder cases, with the antibiotic administered orally, associated with a residue-free diet for 7 days.

Complicated acute diverticulitis will all require hospital admission. In all cases, they will require broad-spectrum antibiotics associated with control of the infectious focus. In cases of intra-abdominal abscesses, control of the focus can be considered by placing a CT-guided percutaneous drainage. If this is not possible or is not effective, surgical drainage should be performed.

In cases of acute peritonitis, surgery is mandatory. Depending on the severity of the patient, the peritoneal contamination, and the size of the perforation, different surgical options can be considered, ranging from resection of the affected colon segment and colostomy (Hartmann technique) to resection of the colon segment and primary anastomosis or even suturing the perforation, washing the abdominal cavity, and placing a drain [1, 5, 6].

11.8 Physical Therapy Options

Possible physical therapy treatments that might be considered for diverticular disease and acute diverticulitis include:

- Working on the pelvic floor muscles: helping to strengthen the pelvic floor muscles.
- Breathing exercises: Deep-breathing techniques can help improve relaxation, decrease pain, and improve peristalsis. Additionally, diaphragmatic breathing can help reduce stress and improve oxygenation, decreasing pain and promoting relaxation.
- Manual therapy techniques: practical mobilization or manipulation of the abdominal region can help relieve pain and improve mobility.
- Determine an exercise table: tailored exercises that focus on general fitness and strength training may be beneficial.
- Relaxation techniques: stress reduction techniques, such as meditation, mindfulness, and progressive muscle relaxation, help manage stress and relieve symptoms associated with diverticulitis.
- Electrotherapy: techniques such as transcutaneous electrical nerve stimulation (TENS) can be used to manage pain. TENS has been shown to be effective in reducing abdominal pain by modulating pain signals.
- -Heat therapy: application of heat packs to the abdomen can help alleviate pain and discomfort by relaxing the muscles and improving blood flow.

It is important to keep in mind that the use of physical therapy treatments for acute diverticulitis should be individualized based on the patient's specific symptoms, needs, and goals. Actually, there is little evidence to support the effectiveness of physical therapy for this pathology [5, 6].

Bibliography

1. Wilkins T, Embry K, George R. Diagnosis and management of acute diverticulitis. Am Fam Physician. 2013;87(9):612–20.
2. Strate LL, Morris AM. Epidemiology, pathophysiology, and treatment of diverticulitis. Gastroenterology. 2019;156(5):1282–1298.e1.
3. Francis NK, Sylla P, Abou-Khalil M, Arolfo S, Berler D, Curtis NJ, et al. EAES and SAGES 2018 consensus conference on acute diverticulitis management: evidence-based recommendations for clinical practice. Surg Endosc. 2019;33(9):2726–41.
4. Jerjen F, Zaidi T, Chan S, Sharma A, Mudliar R, Soomro K, et al. Magnetic resonance imaging for the diagnosis and management of acute colonic diverticulitis: a review of current and future use. J Med Radiat Sci. 2021;68(3):310–9.
5. Roig JV, Sánchez-Guillén L, García-Armengol JJ. Acute diverticulitis and surgical treatment. Minerva Chir. 2018;73(2):163–78.
6. Sánchez-Velázquez P, Grande L, Pera M. Outpatient treatment of uncomplicated diverticulitis: a systematic review. Eur J Gastroenterol Hepatol. 2016;28(6):622–7.

12 Chronic Constipation

Aarón Díaz-Arranz, Miguel Bermejo-Martínez, Miguel Ángel San-Pedro, Marcos González-Martínez, and Ana Martín-Nieto

12.1 Definition

Chronic constipation is a condition presented by certain subjects who have limited ability or extreme difficulty to defecate regularly, in addition to making great over-exertion [1]. It is considered chronic when it lasts over 3 months [1].

Constipation is a common condition that appears in most people at least once in their life but usually lasting for a short period of time and is self-limited. However, chronic constipation can be a major problem and affect negatively the quality of life of people who suffer from it [2].

12.2 Epidemiology

Chronic constipation is a very common disorder, affecting 15% of the world's population. Its prevalence is higher in developed countries, probably due to lifestyle and the type of diet consumed. It affects more frequently to women and elderly over 65 years of age [3].

A. Díaz-Arranz · M. Bermejo-Martínez · M. Á. San-Pedro · M. González-Martínez · A. Martín-Nieto (✉)
San Juan de Dios Foundation, Madrid, Spain

Department of Health Sciences, San Juan de Dios School of Nursing and Physical Therapy, Comillas Pontifical University, Madrid, Spain
e-mail: amartinn@comillas.edu

© The Author(s), under exclusive license to Springer Nature Switzerland AG 2025
J. Ruiz-Tovar, A. Martín-Nieto (eds.), *Physical Therapy for Gastrointestinal Disorders*, https://doi.org/10.1007/978-3-031-83651-0_12

12.3 Etiology

Chronic constipation is a disorder that may be secondary to different causes. First of all, some medications ingested can cause chronic constipation by slowing down intestinal motility. There are some drugs that have a sedative effect on the central nervous system (CNS), causing this to slow down and thus contributing to constipation [1]. Among drugs that can cause chronic constipation are opiates, anticholinergics, diuretics, antidiarrheals, calcium channel blockers, and tricyclic antidepressants [1].

In addition, some pathologies that cause metabolic disturbances such as diabetes mellitus, hypothyroidism, or hypercalcemia can also contribute to the development of chronic constipation.

On the other hand, constipation can be due to mechanical obstruction of the bowel, like in colorectal cancer and intestinal adhesions or with rectocele or strictures at any level of the bowel or the colon [1]. Pathologies related to the CNS can also increase the risk of constipation, as in the case of Parkinson's disease or multiple sclerosis [1].

In addition to these factors, lifestyle plays a fundamental role in the development of chronic constipation, as it has been proven that a low-fiber diet, lacking legumes, fruits, and vegetables, can significantly increase the risk of suffering constipation. A sedentary lifestyle is also a risk factor, as it slows intestinal motility. Finally, not drinking enough water may be a predisposing factor, as the stool may be more difficult to excrete if it is not hydrated [1].

12.4 Pathophysiology

Chronic constipation is a multifaceted disease with diverse underlying pathophysiological mechanisms. The key factors and mechanisms involved in the pathophysiology of chronic constipation are described below. First, it may be caused by altered intestinal motility including possible slow transit or neuromuscular desynchronization. A slower colonic transit prolongs the time that stool remains in the colon. This allows greater absorption of water, making the stool drier and harder [4]. In addition, signals between the brain and the intestine may not be synchronized, affecting the progressive peristalsis and the ability of the colon to move stool efficiently [5]. On the other hand, some pelvic floor dysfunctions may cause constipation; among these alterations may be rectal prolapse or a dysfunction of the puborectalis muscle, which prevents the effective expulsion of feces. Lack of coordination of the muscles involved in defecation can make it difficult to pass stool, despite having an urge to do so. A lack of relaxation or paradoxical contraction of the anal sphincter may also occur during defecation [6].

Finally, there are a number of neurogenic factors that may explain constipation. The nerves that control bowel movement may be damaged or not function properly (as in the case of neurological diseases), which may decrease bowel motility. On the other hand, also some disorders in the autonomic nervous system, which regulates bowel function, may contribute to constipation [7].

12.5 Clinical Manifestations

Among the clinical manifestations associated with constipation are the following [1]:

- Abdominal pain
- Abdominal distention
- Pain during bowel movements
- Presence of meteorism
- Hard, caprine, or macro stools
- Perianal pain during the defecation
- Blood in some occasions, which may appear at the end of the bowel movement or urinary symptoms

In the case of the elderly and vulnerable population, in addition to these manifestations, there may be frequent complications such as "fecal impaction" (occupation of the anal canal and large intestine by hard, compact stool), dilation of the colon, and even volvulus (twisting of a section of the large intestine due to dilation), along with the classic local consequences of defecatory straining and hard stool (hemorrhoids, fissures, and anal prolapse) [8].

12.6 Diagnostic Tests

Clinical history is an essential part of diagnosis; a correct anamnesis must obtain clear data regarding the consistency, shape, caliber, appearance, and frequency of the stool. To make it easier for the patient to describe his stool, the Bristol scale (Table 12.1) is used [9]. Types 1 and 2 of this scale correspond to slow transit (constipation) and types 6 and 7 to accelerated transit (diarrhea).

Rome IV criteria can also be used for diagnosis [10] (Table 12.2).

Table 12.1 Bristol scale

Type	Description
1	Pellets (difficult to expel), slime, or goat feces
2	Hard, dry, cracked, sausage-like appearance
3	With hard sausage appearance and cracks
4	Sausage-like with a smooth, soft surface
5	Smooth pieces with sharp edges (easily ejected)
6	Smooth, unshaped pieces with irregular edges
7	Aqueous, no solid parts, entirely liquid

Table 12.2 Rome IV criteria for the diagnosis of chronic constipation

It must include two or more of the following elements:
(a) Effort in at least 25% of bowel movements (b) Hard bowel movements in at least 25% of bowel movements (c) Feeling of incomplete evacuation in at least 25% of evacuations (d) Sensation of obstruction or anorectal blockage in at least 25% of bowel movements (e) Use of maneuvers to facilitate evacuation at least 25% of the time (digital evacuation, pelvic floor support) (f) Less than three bowel movements per week
Loose bowel movements that occur exceptionally if no laxatives are used
Insufficient criteria for the diagnosis of irritable bowel syndrome
Symptoms present in the last 3 months and with onset at least 6 months before

In addition to the use of different scales and a detailed clinical history of the patient, the use of physiological studies is recommended:

Anorectal manometry: Consists of measuring the pressures in the anal canal and rectum at rest and during defecatory maneuvers. It also allows evaluation of intrinsic and extrinsic anorectal innervation, volume, and sensitivity of the rectum. It is considered indicated in patients who do not respond to treatment with lifestyle changes, bolus-forming agents, osmotic laxatives, and prokinetics [1].

Balloon expulsion test: Consists of introducing a balloon into the rectum that is inflated with air or liquid, and the patient is asked to evacuate it. The balloon should be inflated to a volume that gives the patient the sensation of having to defecate, and the patient will expel the balloon in privacy. The preferred approach is to quantify the time required to expel a rectal balloon in the sitting position (normal values may vary according to technique). It is indicated in patients who do not respond to treatment with lifestyle changes, bolus-forming agents, osmotic laxatives, and prokinetics, in whom constipation is suspected to be caused by impaired defecation [1].

Determination of colonic transit time: Colonic transit time is the time it takes for stool to pass through the colon. It is determined by ingesting small radiopaque contrast and then performing serial plain abdominal X-rays to quantify the time. It is indicated in patients who do not respond to treatment with lifestyle changes, bolus-forming agents, osmotic laxatives, and prokinetics. This test allows the identification of patients who have constipation due to slow colonic transit [1].

Video defecography: It is a type of medical radiological imaging in which the mechanics of a patient's defecation are visualized in real time using a fluoroscope. The anatomy and function of the anorectum and pelvic floor can be dynamically studied at various stages during defecation. It is indicated in rectocele and pelvic floor disorders.

Colonoscopy: In the different clinical practice guidelines, colonoscopy is recommended in those patients who present with constipation and alarming signs and/or symptoms, suspicious of colorectal neoplasms. It is indicated in patients with constipation who do not respond to treatment and in patients over 50 years of age with a family history of colorectal cancer who have not been evaluated by colonoscopy after the onset of constipation [1].

12.7 Conventional Treatment

First of all, it is recommended that patients adopt a series of healthy lifestyle habits and follow these recommendations [11]:

- Intake of foods rich in fiber helps the formation of stool, due to the inability of our body to process fiber.
- Increase water intake: for the correct normal functioning of the physiology of the digestive and excretory system.
- Increase physical exercise to stimulate intestinal motility, favoring the movement of stool and, thus, its correct deposition.
- Do not ignore the need to go to the bathroom.
- Take the necessary time for the deposition.

These types of measures usually work in the early stages, but when constipation is chronic, it must be complemented with adequate pharmacological treatment [11, 12]:

- Bulk formers: such as psyllium, calcium polycarbophils, or methylcellulose; these compounds are responsible for adding bulk to the stool, which also contribute to its softer consistency.
- Stimulants of the intestinal motility: such as bisacodyl and sennosides, which are responsible for promoting intestinal movement, so that an effective mobilization of feces takes place.
- Osmotics: such as oral magnesium, magnesium citrate, lactulose, or polyethylene glycol; these types of laxatives increase the secretion of intestinal fluid, thus helping the passage of stool throughout the intestinal tract.
- Stool softeners: such as docusate sodium or docusate calcium; these are substances that, as their name indicates, soften the stool, facilitating its deposition.
- Peripheral opioid receptor antagonists: because opioid analgesics can cause constipation, substances that inhibit opioid receptors can return the patient to normal. An example could be methylnaltrexone.
- Lubricants: such as those formed by glycerin, among other materials, this type of laxatives is able to lubricate the structures through which the stool will later pass, facilitating its movement to the rectum.

It should be emphasized that, in general, bulk-forming and osmotic laxatives should always be used first, and in more severe cases, stimulant laxatives can be indicated [12].

In addition, if for some reason none of these medications are effective or if the constipation is due to an obstruction, a rectocele, or a constriction, it can be considered to solve this problem surgically, either by solving the obstruction or by removing the affected segment of the colon. Surgical treatment is reserved as a final therapeutic option only for those cases where all pharmacologic treatments have failed and chronic constipation persists with significant effect on the quality of life of the patient [1, 12].

12.8 Physiotherapy Treatment

Chronic constipation can be effectively managed with a variety of physical therapy treatments. The following is a complete overview of physical therapy interventions:

Abdominal massage therapy: Set of manual therapy techniques in which physiotherapy is combined with a massage on the direction of the normal movement of defecation, stimulating the muscles in the area and peristalsis, in turn facilitating normal defecation. Abdominal massage has demonstrated efficacy in the control of chronic functional constipation superior to pharmacological treatment. In addition, abdominal massage can be accompanied with isometric exercises of the abdominal musculature and diaphragmatic breathing exercises [13, 14].

Neuromuscular taping: Neuromuscular taping is a common technique in physical therapy that helps reduce pain, regulates muscle function, and increases circulation. In recent years, neuromuscular taping has been used on internal organs, especially in colorectal and anal problems such as constipation. This improvement is attributed to the effect of the taping on the reflex region of the colon, which may regulate myofascial tone and increase blood flow [15, 16].

Posterior tibial nerve electrical stimulation: Posterior tibial nerve stimulation is a form of neuromodulation that can regulate sphincter function and bowel motility. Electrical stimulation of the posterior tibial nerve can improve symptomatology of patients with chronic constipation as well as reduce the time to defecation [17].

Hypopressive exercises: classified as a series of exercises that help decrease pelvic pressure and increase intestinal peristalsis, they can be a useful tool for chronic constipation caused by pelvic floor dyssynergia [18].

Biofeedback or pelvic floor rehabilitation: Postulated as a technique that is even more effective than the use of laxatives in patients with chronic constipation due to dyssynergia of the pelvic floor. The procedure consists of correcting the contractions of the pelvic floor and anal sphincter, which allows the patient to relax these structures, and, consequently, normal bowel movement [6, 19].

In addition to these specific physical therapy treatments, it is recommended that the practitioner instruct patients on the best posture to improve defecation. Considering the anatomy of the human body and how cavities are oriented, a small elevation of the feet with respect to the floor, as well as a small flexion of the trunk at the time of going to the bathroom, can facilitate the exit of fecal material [12].

Bibliography

1. Neri L, Basilisco G, Corazziari E, Stanghellini V, Bassotti G, Bellini M, et al. Constipation severity is associated with productivity losses and healthcare utilization in patients with chronic constipation. United European Gastroenterol J. 2014;2:138–47.
2. Oh SJ, Fuller G, Patel D, Khalil C, Spalding W, Nag A, et al. Chronic constipation in the United States: results from a population-based survey assessing healthcare seeking and use of pharmacotherapy. Am J Gastroenterol. 2020;115:895–905.
3. Shin JE, Jung HK, Lee TH, Jo Y, Lee H, Song KH, et al. Guidelines for the diagnosis and treatment of chronic functional constipation in Korea. J Neurogastroenterol Motil. 2016;22(3):383–411.
4. Bassotti G, Imbimbo BP, Betti C, Dozzini G, Morelli A. Impaired colonic motor response to eating in patients with slow-transit constipation. Am J Gastroenterol. 1992;87(4):504–8.
5. Lang-Illievich K, Bornemann-Cimenti H. Opioid-induced constipation: a narrative review of therapeutic options in clinical management. Korean J Pain. 2019;32(2):69–78.
6. Skardoon GR, Khera AJ, Emmanuel AV, Burgell RE. Review article: dyssynergic defaecation and biofeedback therapy in the pathophysiology and management of functional constipation. Aliment Pharmacol Ther. 2017;46(4):410–23.
7. El-Salhy M. Chronic idiopathic slow transit constipation: pathophysiology and management. Color Dis. 2003;5(4):288–96.
8. Forootan M, Bagheri N, Darvishi M. Chronic constipation: a review of literature. Medicine. 2018;97(20):e10631.
9. Nightingale JM, Paine P, McLaughlin J, Emmanuel A, Martin JE, Lal S. The management of adult patients with severe chronic small intestinal dysmotility. Gut. 2020;69(12):2074–92.
10. Mearin F, Lacy BE, Chang L, Chey WD, Lembo AJ, Simren M, et al. Bowel disorders. Gastroenterology. 2016;S0016-5085(16):00222–5.
11. Black CJ, Ford AC. Chronic idiopathic constipation in adults: epidemiology, pathophysiology, diagnosis and clinical management. Med J Aust. 2018;209(2):86–91.
12. Barbara G, Barbaro MR, Marasco G, Cremon C. Chronic constipation: from pathophysiology to management. Minerva Gastroenterol. 2023;69(2):277–90.
13. Silva CAG, Motta MEFA. The use of abdominal muscle training, breathing exercises and abdominal massage to treat paediatric chronic functional constipation. Color Dis. 2013;15(5):e250–5.
14. Doğan İG, Gürşen C, Akbayrak T, Balaban YH, Vahabov C, Üzelpasacı E, et al. Abdominal massage in functional chronic constipation: a randomized placebo-controlled trial. Phys Ther. 2022;102(7):pzac058.
15. Morris D, Jones D, Ryan H, Ryan CG. The clinical effects of Kinesio® Tex taping: a systematic review. Physiother Theory Pract. 2013;29(4):259–70.
16. Karaaslan Y, Karakus A, Ogutmen Koc D, Bayrakli A, Toprak Celenay S. Effectiveness of abdominal massage versus Kinesio taping in women with chronic constipation: a randomized controlled trial. J Neurogastroenterol Motil. 2024.; In press.; https://doi.org/10.5056/jnm23131.
17. Hamedfar M, Ghaderi F, Salehi Pourmehr H, Soltani A, Ghojazadeh M, Vahed N. Posterior tibial nerve electrical stimulation in chronic constipation: a systematic review and meta-analysis. Gastroenterol Hepatol Bed Bench. 2024;17(1):6–16.
18. Andromanakos NP, Pinis SI, Kostakis AI. Chronic severe constipation: current pathophysiological aspects, new diagnostic approaches, and therapeutic options. Eur J Gastroenterol Hepatol. 2015;27(3):204–14.
19. Zar-Kessler C, Kuo B, Cole E, Benedix A, Belkind-Gerson J. Benefit of pelvic floor physical therapy in pediatric patients with dyssynergic defecation constipation. Dig Dis. 2019;37(6):478–85.

Fecal Incontinence

13

Sara Ciriza-Torres, Marta García-Ramos, Marta López-Acedo, Celia Rodríguez-Ruano, and Jaime Ruiz-Tovar

13.1 Definition

Fecal incontinence is the involuntary loss of stools, both solid and liquid. According to the Rome III criteria, it can also be defined as the uncontrolled passage of fecal material recurrently for 3 months in people over 4 years old, accompanied by abnormal pelvic floor muscle function, minor sphincter innervation abnormalities, normal or altered bowel habits, and psychological causes. This condition can be caused by muscle injury, nerve injury, diarrhea, loss of rectal storage capacity, anorectal or pelvic surgery, rectal prolapse, or diabetes mellitus, although the most common cause is multifactorial [1].

13.2 Epidemiology

Fecal incontinence affects around 8% of the population, being more common in middle-aged or elderly adults. It is estimated that 15% of people over 70 years old suffer from fecal incontinence, especially affecting women over 60–70 years old, usually due to muscle weakness associated with aging or injuries caused during childbirth [2].

S. Ciriza-Torres · M. García-Ramos · M. López-Acedo · C. Rodríguez-Ruano
J. Ruiz-Tovar (✉)
San Juan de Dios Foundation, Madrid, Spain

Department of Health Sciences, San Juan de Dios School of Nursing and Physical Therapy, Comillas Pontifical University, Madrid, Spain

© The Author(s), under exclusive license to Springer Nature Switzerland AG 2025
J. Ruiz-Tovar, A. Martín-Nieto (eds.), *Physical Therapy for Gastrointestinal Disorders*, https://doi.org/10.1007/978-3-031-83651-0_13

13.3 Etiology

The most common causes of fecal incontinence in adults are [3]:

- Diarrhea: when stool is soft or liquid, as in diarrhea, it easily overcomes the barrier represented by the anus.
- Chronic constipation: causes weakness and stretching of the pelvic floor muscles, allowing soft or watery stool, formed above the hard mass to facilitate its expulsion, to leak through it.
- Nerve injury: the nerves in the anus and rectum respond less intensely to the presence of stool, and the information about anorectal filling does not reach the central nervous system, preventing the transmission of increased pressure information to the anal sphincters to prevent stool leakage.
- Neurological diseases: certain neurological diseases (multiple sclerosis, stroke, Parkinson's, etc.) affect the pelvic nerves, both in sensory reception and motor signal transmission to the pelvic floor muscles, causing fecal incontinence.
- Rectal prolapse: it causes the rectum to descend through the anus and may prevent the muscles around the anus from closing completely, allowing stool leakage.
- Rectocele: incontinence occurs exclusively in women as the rectum protrudes through the vagina.
- Vaginal childbirth: During childbirth, injuries to the anal sphincter may occur. These sometimes go unnoticed and other times are detected and sutured, but the anal sphincter often loses tone. This is possibly the most common cause of incontinence in women and increases with the number of births.
- Anal surgery (hemorrhoids or anal fissure): these surgeries can damage the anal sphincter and leave incontinence as a sequela.

13.4 Physiopathology

Fecal incontinence is caused by various abnormalities in the anorectal area, both anatomical and physiological [4, 5]:

- *Structural alterations:* Damages to the internal anal sphincter can cause incontinence. The most common cause of sphincter injury is obstetric trauma, increasing the risk in multiparous women and instrumental deliveries (forceps or vacuum). Other causes of structural injuries include anorectal surgery and perineal trauma.
- *Rectal alterations:* Rectal hypersensitivity, damage to the wall conformation, and abnormal rectal accommodation are other mechanisms causing fecal incontinence. This can be associated with increased bowel frequency or decreased ability to defer defecation.
- *Functional abnormalities:* Defecation requires the integration of stimuli from the rectal wall, pelvic floor, and anal canal. People with functional abnormalities

often have decreased rectal sensitivity, resulting in stool accumulation in the rectal ampulla and anal canal, which progressively dilate. Factors associated with this sensory alteration are often due to neurological damage, spinal injuries, or the use of certain medications.

13.5 Clinical Assessment

Clinical evaluation is based on anamnesis, physical examination, and the completion of questionnaires [6–8]:

Anamnesis: It should include personal history of systemic diseases and surgical and obstetric history. It should characterize the type of incontinence:

- Urgency incontinence: occurs when there is not enough time to reach the bathroom and continence mechanisms are insufficient to prevent leakage.
- Passive incontinence: occurs when there is loss of feces without the sensation of defecation (occurs in neurological diseases or overflow diarrhea, where the fecal bolus does not trigger the defecation reflex).
- Soiling: presence of liquid stool around the anus or in the underwear.
- Gas incontinence: involuntary escape of gases; very common and limiting.

Physical examination: the main physical examination used is digital rectal exam, where a hypotonic anal sphincter can be appreciated [9, 10].

Questionnaires: these are very helpful in identifying symptoms and the severity of incontinence, as well as the impact on the patient's quality of life. Frequently used questionnaires include [9, 10]:

- Wexner scale: This scale scores from 0 (never) to 4 (always) the incontinence for liquid stool, solid stool, and gases, the use of absorbent materials, and the alteration in quality of life. The final score is the sum of the five items, obtaining a score of 0–20. A Wexner score of 9 or higher indicates a loss of quality of life.
- Defecation diary: Consists of the daily and systematic recording, for at least 2 or 3 weeks, of the most prevalent symptoms of the patient. The results of this continence diary can be divided into three subgroups: mild incontinence if there are less than three episodes of incontinence per week, moderate incontinence if there are between three and ten episodes per week, and severe incontinence if there are more than ten episodes of incontinence.
- Fecal Incontinence Quality of Life Scale (FIQLS): Fecal incontinence is associated with emotional disorders such as loss of self-esteem and limitation in social, work, and sexual activities. The FIQLS questionnaire is a specific quality of life questionnaire applicable to patients with fecal incontinence. It consists of 29 questions that study 4 health domains, lifestyle, behavior, depression, and shame, all associated with incontinence.

13.6 Diagnosis

To confirm the diagnosis, various complementary tests are available [9, 10]:

- Anal manometry: important in evaluating sphincter function, key in studying resting and effort pressure.
- Endoanal ultrasound: the gold standard for evaluating sphincters in fecal incontinence.
- Proctography: X-ray video images that allow us to see the amount of stool the rectum can retain.
- Colonoscopy: used in differential diagnosis with other pathologies that cause anal incontinence, such as colorectal tumors.
- Magnetic resonance imaging: useful in diagnosing multicompartmental alterations, such as pelvic organ prolapses.
- Defecography: dynamic radiological study of anorectal and pelvic floor anatomy and function.
- Neurophysiological studies: Can detect denervations or sensory alterations in apparently idiopathic incontinence.

13.7 Conventional Treatment

Medical treatment for this type of pathology starts with dietary changes to improve and modify any alteration that may appear in intestinal transit (avoiding both diarrheal episodes and fecalomas) [9, 10].

Another tool to combat fecal incontinence is pharmacotherapy. This option is a good way to eradicate this pathology in patients with persistent diarrhea. One of the most used drugs is loperamide, which reduces intestinal peristalsis and increases water absorption from the fecal bolus, making it a firmer mass [9, 10].

As a last resort, surgery can be complex, with its risks and complications. Therefore, patients with fecal incontinence must have a high "score" and a significant alteration in their lifestyle. The operation depends on the characteristics of the incontinence, the integrity of the sphincter apparatus, and the personal characteristics of the patients. Surgical options include sacral root neuromodulation, sphincteroplasty, graciloplasty, or the placement of an artificial anal sphincter, all with variable success rates and not without complications [9, 10].

13.8 Physical Therapy Treatment Options

The main physical therapy approach to treating fecal incontinence will be perineal muscle exercises and biofeedback.

Perineal muscle exercises were described by Kegel in 1950. These exercises are performed to relieve incontinence. They should be done 10 times a day at regular intervals. Kegel demonstrated the relationship between hypotonia or weakness of the perineal muscles and pelvic floor dysfunctions. Symptoms improve significantly or disappear completely with exercises aimed at strengthening these structures. Kegel pioneered the development of the Pelvic Floor Muscle Training System (PFMTS), consisting of a series of exercises designed to increase the contraction strength of the perineal muscles. The effectiveness of this method has been widely proven [10].

This pathology is treated by combining these perineal muscle exercises with another technique known as biofeedback. Biofeedback consists of the application of electrodes in the perineal area. What these electrodes will do is to transform the patient's exercises into information that will be recorded through a graph on a monitor that will be helpful to know if the patient is doing the exercises properly. It involves the collection of information by sensors that capture signals from the somatic nervous system, which transmit voluntary actions from the brain to the muscles. This process records muscle activity using a method known as electromyogram [11]. Biofeedback is indicated for patients with fecal incontinence who do not respond well to conventional treatment since only 60% of patients with fecal incontinence experience long-term improvement [10].

Posterior tibial nerve neurostimulation was first described by Shafik in 2003 [12]. Since then, its use has become standard practice in the treatment of fecal incontinence. It is a simple and highly reproducible technique that does not require anesthesia and can be easily performed in the outpatient clinic. Neuromodulation is applied through a patch (transcutaneous) or by means of a very fine needle (percutaneous) placed posterior to the tibial malleolus. We know that it is getting to stimulate the posterior tibial nerve if sensory response is perceived in the sole of the foot by the patient. It is not necessary to get to notice motor response or pain. There are different regimens of sessions, but the most used is 30 min weekly for 3 months.

Regarding the results, a literature review done in 2018 [13] showed that, in all clinical trials and case series, neurostimulation of the posterior tibial nerve was able to reduce incontinence episodes and increase stool delay. It also improved quality of life and improved the severity of incontinence.

Bibliography

1. Bharucha AE, Knowles CH, Mack I, Malcolm A, Oblizajek N, Rao S, et al. Faecal incontinence in adults. Nat Rev Dis Prim. 2022;8(1):53.
2. Cerdan Santacruz C, Santos Rancano R, Vigara Garcia M, Fernandez Perez C, Ortega Lopez M, Cerdan Miguel J. Prevalence of anal incontinence in a working population within a healthcare environment. Scand J Gastroenterol. 2017;52(12):1340–7.
3. Wald A. Diagnosis and management of fecal incontinence. Curr Gastroenterol Rep. 2018;20(3):94.
4. López-Delgado A, Arroyo A, Ruiz-Tovar J, Alcaide MJ, Diez M, Moya P, et al. Effect on anal pressure of percutaneous posterior tibial nerve stimulation for faecal incontinence. Color Dis. 2014;16(7):533–7.
5. Wald A. Clinical practice. Fecal incontinence in adults. N Engl J Med. 2007;356(16):1648–55.

6. Paquette IM, Varma MG, Kaiser AM, Steele SR, Rafferty JF. The American Society of Colon and Rectal Surgeons' clinical practice guideline for the treatment of fecal incontinence. Dis Colon Rectum. 2015;58(7):623–36.
7. Jiang AC, Panara A, Yan Y, Rao SSC. Assessing anorectal function in constipation and fecal incontinence. Gastroenterol Clin N Am. 2020;49(3):589–606.
8. Moya P, Navarro JM, Arroyo A, López A, Ruiz-Tovar J, Calpena R. Sacral nerve stimulation during pregnancy in patients with severe fecal incontinence. Tech Coloproctol. 2013;17(2):245–6.
9. Carrington EV, Scott SM, Bharucha A, Mion F, Remes-Troche JM, Malcolm A, et al. Expert consensus document: advances in the evaluation of anorectal function. Nat Rev Gastroenterol Hepatol. 2018;15(5):309–23.
10. Bharucha AE. Outcome measures for fecal incontinence: anorectal structure and function. Gastroenterology. 2004;126(1 Suppl 1):90–8.
11. Narayanan SP, Bharucha AE. A practical guide to biofeedback therapy for pelvic floor disorders. Curr Gastroenterol Rep. 2019;21(5):21.
12. Shafik A, Ahmed I, El-Sibai O, Mostafa RM. Percutaneous peripheral neuromodulation in the treatment of fecal incontinence. Eur Surg Res. 2003;35(2):103–7.
13. Arroyo Fernandez R, Avendano Coy J, Ando Lafuente S, Martin Correa Ma T, Ferri Morales A. Posterior tibial nerve stimulation in the treatment of fecal incontinence: a systematic review. Rev Esp Enferm Dig. 2018;110(9):577–88.

Proctalgia Fugax

14

Michelle Carvajal, Xenia Barbú, Angel Martinez,
Jimmy Muñoz, and Jaime Ruiz-Tovar

14.1 Definition

Proctalgia fugax is defined as a sharp, sudden pain that occurs in the anus, lasting from seconds to minutes. The pain is recurrent and often presents a sudden onset. The intensity of the pain can be mild and tolerable, but in several cases, it can be severe and impacts daily life. The pain predominantly appears at night and is capable of awakening the patient, at frequent intervals of less than 30 min. The pain resembles a spasm in the anus.

Proctalgia fugax is considered as a functional rectal pathology, without evidence of tissue damage. Thus, its diagnosis is by exclusion of other pathologies.

It was first described in 1841 by Hall, but actually, there is still little evidence about its physiopathology and treatment [1, 2].

14.2 Epidemiology

Knowing the exact prevalence of this pathology is difficult, as it is not usually reported by the patients who suffer from it. It has been estimated that between 4% and 18% of the population experiences proctalgia fugax, but only about 20% seek medical attention for it, as episodes are infrequent, the average being less than five episodes per year. But it should be noted that sometimes, the frequency is much higher and may occur on a daily basis [3, 4].

This pathology is usually more present in women than in men, and the average age of presentation typically ranges between 30 and 60 years old.

M. Carvajal · X. Barbú · A. Martinez · J. Muñoz · J. Ruiz-Tovar (✉)
San Juan de Dios Foundation, Madrid, Spain

Department of Health Sciences, San Juan de Dios School of Nursing and Physical Therapy, Comillas Pontifical University, Madrid, Spain

© The Author(s), under exclusive license to Springer Nature Switzerland AG 2025

J. Ruiz-Tovar, A. Martín-Nieto (eds.), *Physical Therapy for Gastrointestinal Disorders*, https://doi.org/10.1007/978-3-031-83651-0_14

14.3 Etiology

Its etiology is not clear, and there are different etiological hypothesis, but none provides conclusive evidence.

Its etiopathogenesis is attributed to several causes: spasm of the anal sphincter muscles, hypertrophy of the internal anal sphincter, compression of the pudendal nerve, psychological disorders, allergies, venous stasis, mechanical factors, and infections, although a causal relation has not been clearly established in any case [2, 5].

14.4 Physiopathology

The physiopathology of proctalgia fugax is poorly understood, similar to other functional anal disorders. The short duration of the symptoms, as well as the varied periodicity, with short and infrequent crises being the most common, make it difficult to study this pathology in depth.

If we accept the hypothesis of anal muscle spam or hypertrophy, it has been observed that during acute pain attacks, patients with proctalgia fugax exhibit motor abnormalities in the anal smooth muscle. Although their anorectal pressures are normal at rest, increased anal resting tone and slow-wave amplitude correlate with longer pain duration. Additionally, a rare inherited myopathy of the internal anal sphincter has been associated with this condition [5].

On the other hand, a neuropathy or a nerve compression of the pudendal nerve, which cannot be evidenced by diagnostic tests, has been also hypothesized.

14.5 Clinical Manifestations

The clinical manifestations of proctalgia fugax show an interindividual variability. However, the most common features of the pain are sensation of tightness or spasm in the muscles of the anal area; episodes of intense pain lasting minutes; nocturnal pain; pain that may radiate to the lower back, genitals, or lower abdomen; episodes of pain occurring spontaneously or due to certain factors such as stress, physical contact, or defecation; and absence of symptoms between episodes [5].

14.6 Diagnosis

The diagnosis of proctalgia fugax is an exclusion diagnosis, made by ruling out other causes of pain. Physical examination, rectoscopy, and anoscopy are normally done in patients who suffer from it, as well as endoanal ultrasound. In certain cases, hypertrophy of the internal anal sphincter can be observed by endoanal ultrasonography [5].

In differential diagnosis, anorectal and pelvic pathologies, ischemia, anal fissures, inflammatory bowel disease, prostatitis, structural alterations of the pelvic floor, perianal abscess, and levator syndrome must be included [6].

14.7 Conventional Treatment

The first recommended treatment for proctalgia fugax is hygienic measures, including warm sitz baths, mostly before going to bed, as proctalgia appears more frequently at night [6–8].

Pharmacological treatment has been useful in several cases, including inhalation of salbutamol and topical nitroglycerine or nifedipine ointments [8, 9]. In persistent cases, local anesthetic blocks, clonidine, or Botox injections can be considered after clarification of risk and benefit. Botulinum A toxin injection can reduce internal anal sphincter pressure, leading to relief of symptoms, and seems a promising option with minimal morbidity in cases of proctalgia fugax that do not respond to other current treatments [10].

In cases where internal anal sphincter hypertrophy is identified, surgical options, such as internal sphincterotomy, may benefit the patient. Sacral nerve stimulation is done in patients who do not respond to other treatments. Electrical stimulation has been shown to reduce inflammation of the levator ani, unspecified functional anorectal pain, anorectal pain, and unspecified functional anorectal and pelvic floor muscle pain [4].

14.8 Physiotherapy Treatment Options

The most effective treatment at present is biofeedback, which consists of a technique that measures human bodily functions, providing helpful information to train the desired musculature and thus to control them. The technique used for proctalgia is videofeedback, which consists in reeducation of the pelvic floor through an electrode that is introduced at the anal or vaginal level, depending on the sex, and thus an interaction with the above mentioned musculature is performed. This will allow voluntary contraction when the machine requests its activation and no contraction when it is not needed [1, 9].

Additionally, there are other treatments aimed to relieve muscle spasm, including massage and pressure on the pelvic floor to relieve anal spasm. Stretching by bringing the knees to the chest, "happy baby pose," might also be useful to relieve pain. In this position, the hands are placed on the buttocks to try to force them apart while putting pressure as if wanting to expel intestinal gas.

Deep-breathing exercises for pelvic floor relaxation have been also reported as therapeutic options [8, 9].

Although not directly related to proctalgia fugax, tibial nerve stimulation (PTNS) has been explored for various pelvic symptoms. PTNS modulates the sacral nerve and has been successfully used to improve symptoms like urinary incontinence, fecal incontinence, constipation, and chronic pelvic pain, including functional anorectal pain. Several authors have reported that the mechanism of action of PTNS is somehow similar to sacral nerve stimulation. As sacral nerve stimulation has been useful in several cases of proctalgia fugax, PTNS appears to be a less invasive therapeutic alternative [11].

References

1. Doggweiler R, Whitmore KE, Meijlink JM, et al. A standard for terminology in chronic pelvic pain syndromes: a report from the chronic pelvic pain working group of the International Continence Society. Neurourol Urodyn. 2017;36:984–1008.
2. Siqueira-Campos VM, de Deus MS, Poli-Neto OB, Rosa-E-Silva JC, de Deus JM, Conde DM. Current challenges in the management of chronic pelvic pain in women: from bench to bedside. Int J Women's Health. 2022;14:225–44.
3. Jeyarajah S, Purkayastha S. Proctalgia fugax. CMAJ. 2013;185:417.
4. Pinto L, Soutinho M, Coutinho Fernandes M, Táboas MI, Leal J, Tomé S, et al. Chronic primary pelvic pain syndromes in women: a comprehensive review. Cureus. 2024;16(12):e74918.
5. Cohee MW, Hurff A, Gazewood JD. Benign anorectal conditions: evaluation and management. Am Fam Physician. 2020;101:24–33.
6. Carrington EV, Popa SL, Chiarioni G. Proctalgia syndromes: update in diagnosis and management. Curr Gastroenterol Rep. 2020;22:35.
7. Chiarioni G, Asteria C, Whitehead WE. Chronic proctalgia and chronic pelvic pain syndromes: new etiologic insights and treatment options. World J Gastroenterol. 2011;17:4447–55.
8. Hawkey A, Chalmers KJ, Micheal S, Diezel H, Armour M. "A day-to-day struggle": a comparative qualitative study on experiences of women with endometriosis and chronic pelvic pain. Fem Psychol. 2022;32:482–500.
9. Jeyarajah S, Chow A, Ziprin P, Tilney H, Purkayastha S. Proctalgia fugax, an evidence based management pathway. Int J Color Dis. 2010;25:1037–46.
10. Grigoriou M, Ioannidis A, Kofina K, Efthimiadis C. Use of botulinum A toxin for proctalgia fugax-a case report of successful treatment. J Surg Case Rep. 2017;2017(11):236.
11. Takano S, Arakawa H. Bilateral posterior tibial nerve stimulation for functional anorectal pain—short term outcome. Int J Color Dis. 2016;31:1053–4.

Obstructive Defecation Syndrome: Anismus and Hirschsprung's Disease

15

Javier Gómez, Roberto Agustín Muñoz, Marco González, and Jaime Ruiz-Tovar

15.1 Definition

Obstructive defecation syndrome consists of the difficulty and impossibility of satisfactorily evacuating the rectum, maintaining the normal defecatory desire in some patients, but lacking it in others [1].

15.2 Etiology

Obstructive defecation syndrome can have several causes. The first of them would be muscular dysfunctions. Within these, we should differentiate between dysfunctions of the striated musculature, as occurs in the anismus, and dysfunctions of the smooth musculature, as occurs in Hirschsprung's disease.

It may be also secondary to sensory dysfunctions characterized by the absence of defecatory desire and is observed more frequently in patients after hysterectomies or after rectal prolapse surgeries, presumably by denervation, although they can also occur in patients without previous surgeries.

Finally, dysfunctions of mechanical or anatomical cause may also occur. In these cases, rather than a mechanical blockage of stool outflow, what occurs is an alteration of the expulsive force vector in the pelvis, as occurs with rectocele and some rectal prolapses [1, 2].

J. Gómez · R. A. Muñoz · M. González · J. Ruiz-Tovar (✉)
San Juan de Dios Foundation, Madrid, Spain

Department of Health Sciences, San Juan de Dios School of Nursing and Physical Therapy, Comillas Pontifical University, Madrid, Spain

© The Author(s), under exclusive license to Springer Nature Switzerland AG 2025

J. Ruiz-Tovar, A. Martín-Nieto (eds.), *Physical Therapy for Gastrointestinal Disorders*, https://doi.org/10.1007/978-3-031-83651-0_15

15.3 Clinical Manifestations

Typical symptoms of obstructive defecation syndrome are difficult rectal evacuation with prolonged defecatory straining, sensation of incomplete evacuation, desire to repeat bowel movements with some degree of defecatory urgency, perineal heaviness, sensation of anal outlet blockage, and self-digitization, which consists of manually removing stool from the anus.

Frequently, obstructive defecation syndrome is associated with psychoneurotic and autonomic symptoms, mainly anxiety and depression [1–3].

15.4 Diagnosis

For a diagnosis of obstructive defecation syndrome, patients must have two or more of the above symptoms in at least 25% of the bowel movements during the last 3 months and for at least 6 months.

In addition to symptomatic criteria, there should also be defecographic evidence of voiding difficulty or impossibly. In rectal manometry, there should be inappropriate contraction of the external anal sphincter or puborectalis muscle, as well as inadequate rectal propulsive force [1–3].

15.5 Treatment

The initial treatment of obstructive defecation syndrome should be conservative and includes a diet rich in fiber, adequate hydration, physical exercise, and the use of enemas or laxatives to promote defecation of stool in a more favorable way.

The most used surgical treatment is sacral root neuromodulation, which has proven to be an effective, minimally invasive, and reversible procedure. In extreme cases in which symptoms cannot be controlled, it may be necessary to perform a colostomy [2–4].

15.6 Physical Therapy Treatment Options

Biofeedback is a well-regarded treatment for obstructive defecation syndrome (ODS), aiming to improve improper muscle coordination. Biofeedback therapy involves using visual or auditory feedback to help patients learn to control their pelvic floor muscles and anal sphincter, often done through manometry or electromyography, which measures muscle activity. Studies have shown that biofeedback can significantly improve symptoms in more than 70% of patients with ODS. It helps patients increase intra-abdominal pressure and relax the anal sphincter during defecation. The therapy typically involves multiple sessions, where patients receive real-time feedback on their muscle activity, allowing them to adjust and improve their defecation technique. However, success with biofeedback largely depends on patient motivation and adherence to the treatment plan [4].

Posterior tibial nerve stimulation (PTNS) is an emerging treatment option for obstructive defecation syndrome (ODS). PTNS involves stimulating the posterior tibial nerve near the ankle using a fine needle and mild electrical impulses. This nerve is connected to the sacral nerve plexus, whose efferent pathway is the pudendal nerve, which influences pelvic floor function. Studies have shown that PTNS can improve symptoms of pelvic floor dysfunction, including ODS. It helps by modulating nerve activity, which can enhance muscle coordination and bowel function. The treatment typically involves weekly sessions over several weeks. It can be a good option for patients who do not respond well to biofeedback or other conservative therapies [5].

15.7 Anismus

Voluntary contraction of the abdominal wall that increases intra-abdominal pressure and synchronous and coordinated voluntary relaxation of the pelvic floor striated musculature are the two basic movements that allow defecation. Lack of coordination of these maneuvers results in a lack of relaxation and inappropriate contraction of the pelvic musculature, followed by increase in intra-abdominal pressure. This lack of relaxation hinders evacuation.

Anismus is more frequent in patients who, due to personal or social inhibition, ignore the normal defecatory desire and turn the postponement of bowel movements into a habit.

Lack of relaxation or contraction of the puborectalis muscle when the patient is asked to make a defecatory effort during physical examination suggests the diagnosis of anismus. Defecographic findings are an insufficient increase or even sharpening of the anorectal angle during straining and an anal opening of less than 1 centimeter with incomplete rectal emptying [6].

15.8 Hirschsprung's Disease (HD)

Hirschsprung's disease is a congenital condition that affects the colon and causes problems with defecation. It occurs due to the absence of nerve cells in parts of the colon, which are essential for stimulating muscle contractions that make stool progress through the colon.

Common symptoms include a swollen belly, vomiting, constipation, and failure to pass the meconium within 48 h after birth.

The exact cause is unknown, but it is often associated with genetic mutations and can run in families.

Diagnosis typically involves physical examination, imaging tests like barium enema, and colonoscopy with biopsy to confirm the absence of nerve cells. The primary treatment is surgery to remove the affected portion of the colon, sometimes even the entire colon [7].

Physical therapy is not a primary treatment for Hirschsprung's disease, but it can play a supportive role in managing symptoms and improving quality of life, especially after surgery. After surgery, physical therapy can help strengthen abdominal and pelvic muscles, which can improve bowel function and reduce discomfort. Pelvic floor exercises help improve bowel control and reduce symptoms like constipation and incontinence. They focus on strengthening the muscles that support the bladder and bowel. Proper breathing techniques can help manage pain and improve overall relaxation, which can be beneficial during recovery.

References

1. Crosby EC, Husk KE. Defecatory dysfunction. Obstet Gynecol Clin N Am. 2021;48(3):653–63.
2. Gold DM, Swash M, Farag A, Ding S, Santoro G, Dodi G. A brief physiology and pathophysiology of the anorectum based on the Integral Theory paradigm. Ann Transl Med. 2024;12(2):25.
3. Desprez C, Bridoux V, Leroi A-M. Disorders of anorectal motility: functional defecation disorders and fecal incontinence. J Visc Surg. 2022;159(1):S40–50.
4. Heinrich H. Deconstructing obstructive defecation syndrome with adaptive biofeedback. Dig Dis Sci. 2022;67:1095–6.
5. Hodgson R, Wagenlehner F, Del Amo E, Inoue H, Abendstein B. Descending perineal syndrome cure by deep transversus perinei ligament repair: surgical options. Ann Transl Med. 2024;12(2):32.
6. Chaudhry Z, Tarnay C. Descending perineum syndrome: a review of the presentation, diagnosis, and management. Int Urogynecol J. 2016;27:1149–56.
7. O'Donnell AM. Translational research in Hirschsprung's disease at the National Children's Research Centre in Dublin. Pediatr Surg Int. 2022;39:33.

MIX
Papier aus verantwortungsvollen Quellen
Paper from responsible sources
FSC® C105338

If you have any concerns about our products,
you can contact us on
ProductSafety@springernature.com

In case Publisher is established outside the EU,
the EU authorized representative is:
Springer Nature Customer Service Center GmbH
Europaplatz 3, 69115 Heidelberg, Germany

Printed by Libri Plureos GmbH
in Hamburg, Germany